65 SIMPLE TIPS FOR A HEALTHY LIFESTYLE

Weight Loss, Exercise, and Healthy Eating

Lewis Demilade Babatope

CONTENTS

INTRODUCTION

"65 Simple Tips for a Healthy Lifestyle" provides the knowledge you need to achieve and maintain a healthy lifestyle. Can you relate to the daily struggle of trying to eat healthy and stay fit?, if so, this book is for you. It gives you the knowledge you need to maintain good health and prevent diseases.

It is a simple fact that, if you are to lose weight, you need to use up more calories than you take in. Maintaining a proper diet can seem like a challenging task, yet it is an important part of a healthy living plan. Eating nutrient-dense foods in their natural state is a key factor in maintaining optimal wellness. Do you ever drive past the gym and wonder if working out is really worth the effort? Exercise offers truly life-changing results if you're willing to put in the effort required.

Are you ready for your transformation? Do not let life pass you by, learn to control it and live it like you are meant to! Remember, this is the only body you have.

ABOUT THE AUTHOR

Lewis Demilade Babatope, the author of **"65 Simple Tips for a Healthy Lifestyle"** founded the website "www.myhealthfuldiet.com" He is a firm believer in helping people quit their inactive and unhealthy lifestyle.

He promotes concepts of health and wellness to people struggling to make a permanent lifestyle change. He also offers readers with strategies and tips needed to turn their lives around by maintaining a healthy diet and exercise routine - two important things needed to live a long and prosperous life. His aim is to provide the resources needed to prevent diseases.

His book and website are his ways of helping people fight the urge to live an unhealthy lifestyle. He has compiled his years of knowledge on various health and fitness topics in his book and website to provide the ultimate resources needed to bring a much awaited transformation.

DISCLAIMER

The information contained in this book is for educational purpose only. The purpose of this book is to promote the understanding of various diet and fitness topics. It is not intended to be a substitute for professional medical advice, diagnosis or treatment.

Always seek the advice of your physician or other qualified health care provider with any questions you may have regarding a medical condition or treatment before undertaking a new health regimen, and never disregard professional medical advice or delay seeking it because of what you read in this book.

PART A: WEIGHT LOSS TIPS

Is the lack of motivation keeping you from losing weight? This section will provide you with the weight loss tips that you can add into your busy schedule.

TIP #1: FIVE EFFECTIVE WEIGHT LOSS ADVICE

It can be very difficult to lose weight, especially if you are left to struggle on your own. Only people who have been unsuccessful on several occasions truly understand how hard it can be to shed those extra pounds. Achieving a slender body also becomes harder with age, but it is achievable. Many of us only discover the incredible secrets later in life.

You will not be the first person who has sought to find a short cut or a miracle product that promises to deliver rapid weight loss. Many dietary supplements are not approved by the Federal Drugs Administration (FDA), so it is hardly surprising to discover that they may be detrimental to your health. Losing excess weight takes time, discipline and effort.

If you want to reduce body fat and build your self esteem, you are going to need to change your lifestyle. On the plus side, if you manage to make the necessary adjustments, you will benefit in more ways than you ever considered possible. Instead of looking for some quick fixes or short cuts, follow some of these simple weight reduction tips.

Healthy, Regular Eating
It may be a saying, but we are what we eat. One of the reasons that we choose to eat healthy meals is because we want to live a longer, fuller life. However, consuming too many carbohydrates will make shedding those excess pounds more difficult. Reduce the amount of breads and pastas that you consume and switch to eating more white meats.

If you eat more grams of protein, this will help you in your other endeavours, such as training at the gym. It is a well-known fact that building some extra muscle means that you will burn more calories. Even if this is not your goal, there is a further benefit. Your body does not convert protein into body fat nearly as quickly as it does carbs.

A further key to keeping your metabolic rate optimized is eating small, regular meals. Rather than eating three 500-calorie meals, try eating five 300-calorie meals. If you also avoid eating late in the evening, this will accelerate your rate of weight loss. Your body converts a higher percentage of calories into fat when you eat later at night.

Watch What You Drink

Stay away from carbonated beverages because they pile on the pounds and are bad for your health. Drink plenty of water because this will help your body to flush out the toxins associated with the burning of fat. The Institute of Medicine believe that men and women should drink 2.2 and 3 liters of water each day, respectively.

Alcohol is another drink that you should give up or reduce. It has 7 calories in every gram and has no nutrients. You may find it easier to sleep at night, but it will result in a poor night's sleep that will leave you feeling famished the next day. If you are finding it hard to quit, consider switching to a glass of red wine every couple of days.

Take a Break from Dieting

Although losing weight takes mental discipline and consistency, there is no harm in taking a day off every now and again. There will be foods that you actively crave, so give yourself some time to eat the foods that you like. All that you have got to do is calculate how many calories are in the serving so that you do not exceed your daily target.

Alternatively, you could try burning off the extra calories at the gym. Almost all cardiovascular machines have a calorie counter; it is easy to determine how much work you need to do to get yourself back on track. However, you do need to remember that it is a lot easier to consume extra calories than it is to burn them off, so do not over do it.

Exercise Regularly

Engaging in exercise that elevates your heart rate is fundamental to losing the pounds. One of the most effective ways of ensuring that you get enough exercise is by joining a gym. If you want to make sure that you train regularly and with the correct amount of intensity, either take a committed friend or hire a personal trainer.

Only you will know whether you are a morning or evening person. You need to train or go to the gym when you feel most passionate. Going to the gym before work will help to oxygenize your blood and give you extra energy. If you go in the evening, it will help to relieve any stress and anxiety that you have experienced over the course of the day.

You need a regular routine, but you must gradually build up your level of intensity. If you have not exercised in a long time, you should get a full health check up by a doctor.

Best Weight Loss Products

Despite the fact that weight loss is predominantly a matter of personal discipline, there are some supplements that will expedite the process. The problem is that it can be difficult to decide which one to take because there are literally thousands of alternatives. While some are clinically proven, others are an elaborate marketing scam.

If you want to find a product that works for you, it is advisable to avoid the ones that promise the improbable. If you are reading claims about how a person has lost 50 pounds in a week and still ate what he liked, it is very unlikely to be true. Instead, identify supplements that are clinically proven and backed by extensive trials.

TIP #2: EIGHT SPICES THAT AID IN WEIGHT LOSS

Herbs and spices allow people to enhance the flavor and variety in their food; however, there is an abundance of scientific data that reveals that herbs and spices have the capacity to do far more than improve taste. The truth is that herbs and spices are rich with anti-oxidants, vitamins, minerals and numerous other medicinal properties that serve to enhance the health and biological functions of humans.

Among these healthy herbs and spices are those that possess the capacity to assist people with their quest to lose weight and effectively manage their weight. The following is a list of herbs and spices that function in a number of different ways to help individuals maintain a healthy body weight through promoting healthy weight loss and prohibiting fat buildup.

1. Ginseng

The metabolism and energy enhancing properties of ginseng are almost legendary. In addition to ginseng's ability to speed up the body's metabolism and boost energy levels, Panax ginseng also has the ability to enhance insulin sensitivity, which increasingly becoming a significant health issue. Consuming ginseng on a daily basis will not only help with weight loss, but it will also help manage blood glucose levels as insulin sensitivity increases.

2. Cayenne Pepper

The active ingredient in cayenne pepper that contributes to weight loss is capsaicin, which is the ingredient that gives all peppers their heat. According to studies, capsaicin performs a number of different functions that serve to assist in the process of weight loss, including shrinking fat tissue, reducing caloric intake, lowering blood fat levels, and fighting the buildup of fat through triggering advantageous protein transformations in the body.

One of the primary benefits of capsaicin is the fact that its ability to produce heat qualifies it as a thermogenic agent, which serves as a catalyst in creating a temporary increase in thermogenic activity in the body. Thermogenesis is the biological process in which the body burns fat in order to generate heat, beneficially impacting the metabolism and fat storage. There is research that suggests that the consumption of thermogenic ingredients has the capacity to raise the body's metabolism by as much as five percent -- increasing fat burning by approximately 16 percent. Cayenne pepper may potentially be able to counteract the natural decrease in the metabolic rate when the body begins to lose weight.

3. Cinnamon

In many areas of the world, cinnamon is considered a wonder spice, based on all of the health benefits it provides. Not only does cinnamon help to boost the body's metabolic rate, but it also has the capacity to assist the body in regulating blood sugar levels. This makes it an ideal option for seasoning for people who are suffering with pre-diabetes or diabetes. Among the benefits of cinnamon consumption are lowered LDL cholesterol, lowered overall cholesterol levels, reduced triglyceride levels, as well as an increased glucose metabolism at a rate of 20 times the normal rate -- significantly improving the ability of the body to properly regulate sugar.

4. Black Pepper

The ingredient that provides black pepper with its powerful and pungent flavor, piperine, also has a number of other benefits that make this spice essential to sustaining optimal health. In addition to providing the flavor of black pepper, piperine also works to block the formation of new fat cells. When black pepper is combined with cayenne pepper and other ingredients, it has the capacity to burn as many calories as a brisk 20-minute walk.

As an additional benefit, black pepper also works to increase the bioavailability of virtually every other herb, spice or food, making it great for preparing every meal.

5. Mustard

It is a little-known fact that mustard is actually a part of the cruciferous vegetable family, along with cabbage, Brussels sprouts and broccoli. When it comes to weight loss, mustard seeds have a powerful impact, possessing the capacity to increase the body's metabolic rate by as much as 20 percent, ensuring that a person will be able to burn calories in a more efficient manner. In fact, as little as three-fifths of a tablespoon of mustard seeds can help a person burn an additional 45 calories per hour.

6. Turmeric

Turmeric is the primacy seasoning that is used in preparing curry dishes. It is the seasoning that provides the yellow-orange coloring in curry dishes; however, turmeric does much more than provide a unique taste, it has a number of medicinal properties. Actually, it is curcumin, the active ingredient in turmeric, which provides the majority of its health benefits. Curcumin helps to block the formation of fat tissue in the body by suppressing the blood vessels that are necessary to form the tissue. This is one way that turmeric contributes to a lower body fat percentage.

7. Ginger

Ginger is a warming spice that is known for its anti-inflammatory properties, and it has also been proven to relax and soothe

the intestinal tract. There is significant research that suggests that ginger also possesses some rather powerful thermogenic properties, meaning that it has the capacity to help boost the body's metabolic rate. Additionally, ginger also has an appetite-suppressant effect when it is consumed, helping to manage food consumption.

8. Cumin

Cumin is another spice that has multiple properties that allow it to positively impact the weight loss and weight management processes. First of all, it has the ability to increase energy production, and it also has the capacity to improve the body's ability to maintain glycemic control, especially with individuals who are suffering with type 2 diabetes. Additionally, ginger aids in the digestive process, which can also enhance the metabolic rate of the body. This is one of those spices that has a substantial history of medicinal use, also being used to enhance memory and provide anti-stress benefits.

The spices listed here have a proven track record in aiding in the weight loss process. When the other benefits that are associated with these spices are considered, it is easy to see why they are so highly recommended by natural medicine practitioners.

TIP #3: FIVE FOODS THAT CAN HELP WEIGHT LOSS

Too often, people fixate on what cannot be eaten when they are trying to lose weight. That's a negative view because there are some foods that can be very useful when it comes to dieting. Here are five interesting - and possibly unexpected - foods that you might want to think about including in your meal plans when you want to lose a few pounds.

Dark chocolate

Forbidden fruits definitely taste sweeter, and people often have cravings when they are on a diet. The good news is that if you crave chocolate, dark chocolate can actually help you lose weight. According to research, dark chocolate can regulate blood sugar spikes and help you to control hunger. Also, dark chocolate is helpful when it comes to managing cravings for sweet and salty food. However, like all high calorie foods, it should only be consumed in moderation.

Beans

Eating beans as part of your diet can help you to feel fuller for longer and therefore naturally reduce your food intake. Beans contain proteins that help to prevent spikes in blood sugar levels. And beans contain plenty of fiber to help you feel full and get your digestive system working well. If you want to lose weight, include beans in your eating plan on a regular basis.

Salads

It's a good idea to start lunch and/or dinner with a salad, like they do in Mediterranean countries. This cuts down on your food intake, since the salad will take the edge off your appetite. Also, it extends meal times, which helps to achieve that full feeling without consuming too many calories. However remember to take salad dressings into account. A healthy option - again chosen by Mediterranean people - is to drizzle a little olive oil over the salad. Alternatively, use a low-calorie, store-bought dressing, or make your own.

Green tea
Green tea contains polyphenols called catechins, which help with digestion and boost the metabolism, leading to an increase in the fat burning which is necessary for weight loss. Additionally green tea can also help in lowering blood cholesterol levels. Green tea is high in antioxidant content, so it's great for general health, as well as being helpful for weight loss.

Grapefruit
Contrary to some claims, grapefruit does not actually boost the metabolism and aid with fat burning. However, it is high in soluble fiber, so eating half a grapefruit before meals could reduce the amount of food you eat, since it takes the edge of your appetite and helps you to stay fuller for longer. Also, the high levels of pectin in grapefruit help to lower blood cholesterol levels, so it's a healthy addition to the diet.

Losing weight is not easy, as you need to make long term changes to your lifestyle. One of those areas that needs to change is your eating pattern. Happily there are some foods that can actually be useful when it comes to losing weight. Seek out those foods and incorporate them into your diet and those excess pounds will soon disappear.

TIP #4: FIVE WAYS TO LOSE WEIGHT WHILE STAYING BUSY

The problem with weight loss is that most people think it takes time. Time is something most people can't afford to spend away from work. Maybe it's a small business or maybe they just have a high pressure job. The point is that they can't think of a way to stay on point career-wise while simultaneously losing weight. Fortunately, there are ways of losing weight without having to cut valuable time away from work.

Stop Eating So Much

The simplest answer is often the best. In this case, the simplest answer is to eat less. If you're gaining weight, that means you're actually not using up all the energy you're consuming. The moment you're not hungry, the moment that you're full, stop eating. Sure, eating is fun. People can eat for pleasure. However, if you're trying to lose weight, you can't do that every time you pick up your spoon and fork.

Get Clear on Why You Want to Lose Weight

Just like getting rich, losing weight is a goal that requires real motivation behind it. You're going to want a real reason, something solid. It has to be more than vanity. There's nothing wrong with losing weight to look good. The problem is that for most people, looking good isn't enough motivation to keep whatever weight they lose off.

Stick to Water

A lot of what gets people to put on the pounds is actually in what they drink, rather than what they eat. Lattes, energy drinks, and sodas – these and more inject a lot of sugar into your diet. These drinks will put a crimp into your weight loss efforts. Even people who can afford to spend days exercising will avoid soft drinks. That's how bad they are for your diet. Stick to water.

Get Rid of the White Bread

If there is anything here that is a shortcut, it's cutting out white bread. White bread is terrible for you. It is almost as bad as drinking sodas daily. White bread does two things for you when you eat it. It fills your stomach and it makes you fat. You'll lose a lot of weight simply by avoiding white bread like the plague.

Don't Snack Around

The good news is that for the most part, food is abundant and readily available. The bad news is that food is abundant and readily available. Anytime you want, you could get a burger and a soda. You could look in the cupboards and find food. Take a look at your life and think about how much snacking you do. Once you work that out, you'll realize just how much extra food you're consuming simply because you're used to eating at certain points of the day.

Being busy doesn't mean you can't lose weight. It just means that you'll have to go with what is necessary, rather than ideal. Cutting out sodas and white bread might not be ideal, but it is completely necessary if you want to lose weight without spending less time at work. If you really want to lose weight, you will do what needs to be done.

TIP #5: FIVE REASONS WHY YOU'RE EXERCISING AND NOT LOSING WEIGHT

Have you ever had this problem? You're exercising regularly, both strength training and aerobic exercise, but you're not losing weight. Even worse, you might be gaining weight despite your regular exercise sessions. You started exercising to shed those extra pounds of body fat, and they aren't coming off. You might wonder why your efforts aren't paying off. Don't worry! It's a common problem, and the lack of weight loss is usually due to one of several possibilities. Let's look at why the number on the scale isn't budging, and what you can do about it.

You're Losing Body Fat and Gaining Muscle
Stepping on a standard bathroom scale gives incomplete information. These scales measure total body weight, weight due to fat, muscle, and bone, plus the fluid in your body. If you're strength training, you could be gaining muscle (which weighs more than fat) while losing body fat. In this case, your body composition is improving, but the change isn't reflected in your weigh-ins. Your weight is increasing, but it's for the right reasons; you're developing a healthier body composition.

Is there an alternative? You could invest in a body scale to measure your body fat percentage. Although these scales aren't entirely accurate, they're helpful for monitoring changes. The key to getting more accurate readings is to step on a body fat scale first thing in the morning after urinating. Make sure your feet are dry too.

If you won't want to invest in a body fat scale, pay attention to how your clothes fit, and monitor the size of your waistline as a marker that you're losing body fat. The scale is only one piece of information.

You're Outeating Your Workouts

Studies show that people sometimes gain weight when they start exercising because they eat more. Research is mixed on this. Some studies even show that exercise suppresses appetite, but there are many factors that can impact the results - exercise intensity, whether you're overweight, gender, age etc.

Still, people often overestimate how many calories they burned during a sweat session and eat accordingly. There's also the "reward" mentality. You burned 300 calories (or so you thought) doing a tough workout, and now you deserve that brownie.

The reality? You burned fewer than 300 calories and that brownie contains more calories than you think. A study by researchers at the University of Ottawa found that people who ate on the basis of the calories they believed they burned consumed two to three times more than they should have.

You're Sitting Too Much after Your Workouts

After a tough workout, you deserve to rest and recover, but sitting for 6 hours in a chair is overkill. That's what many people do when they work a job, and it's not beneficial for their waistline. Sitting also reduces insulin sensitivity, which is bad for your metabolic health.

Doing an exhausting workout sounds like a positive, but if your exercise sessions drain you for the rest of the day, the lack of physical activity throughout the day may more than compensate for the calories you burned during your workout.

For your health, it's important to keep moving throughout the day and avoid the health risks of too much sitting. If you work a desk job, walk around and stretch every 20 to 30 minutes. Try to move more throughout the day, even after your workout.

You're Not Focusing Enough on Good Nutrition

Exercise is a calorie burner, and it improves body composition, but for weight loss, nutrition is at least 80% of the equation. Even the best-laid exercise plans won't lead to weight loss if you ignore the nutrition side of the equation. It's difficult to burn off enough calories through exercise to give you freedom to eat whatever you want. It doesn't work that way.

Don't over restrict calories. Instead, work on improving the composition of what you eat. If you're drinking sugary sports drinks, eating a doughnut as your post-workout snack, and eating junk food because you think exercise allows you to do that, you won't get the results you expect from your exercise sessions. Exercise and nutrition are both important for getting fitter and leaner.

You're Not Giving Your Body Enough Recovery Time

Some people believe that if they exercise, they must give every session maximum effort. So, they work out to exhaustion without giving their body a chance to recover. If you do this consistently, you can elevate cortisol, a stress hormone, that causes gains in belly fat and breakdown of muscle and bone tissue. Too much cortisol harms your physique and health, as it also disrupts your immune system and can affect fertility. It's okay to be passionate but give your body a chance to recover after intense exercise sessions. Balance intense exercise sessions with lighter forms of exercise that relax the mind, like yoga, Tai Chi, stretching, or a walk in nature.

The Bottom Line

Patience is also a virtue. Losing weight takes time. You won't be down 5 pounds after your first week of working out, but each exercise session is doing good things for your mental and physical health. Exercise does more than burn calories; it'll help you stay fit, functional, and healthy. Keep at it!

TIP #6: FOUR FILLING MEALS FOR EFFORTLESS WEIGHT LOSS

There is a fair bit of uninspired, 'chicken and broccoli' type meal plans still circulating in the 'healthy eating' world, so you would be forgiven for thinking that losing fat means sacrificing flavor and fullness for bland, low-calorie alternatives. Luckily, this could not be further from the truth. With a bit of creativity and effort, you can find a ton of tasty, nutrient-dense meal options that leave you feeling full without packing on the extra pounds. But if you are new to the world of diet hacking and unsure where to begin, here are four simple dishes you can try out.

Peanut Butter and Oat Protein Shake
First on the list is a super simple blend of household staples (minus the protein powder, of course). Take two tablespoons of your favorite peanut butter brand, a cup of raw or cooked oats, one cup of your choice of milk (almond, coconut, skimmed, etc.), and a scoop of protein powder, and throw them all in a blender or shaker. Make sure to blend/shake for at least a minute before serving. All these ingredients rank very high on the satiety index and would be more than enough on their own to keep you satisfied, but combining them all into a shake is a surefire way to stay full throughout the day. Peanut butter and oat protein shakes are delicious, filling, and jam-packed with essential macro and micronutrients, including protein, carbs, healthy fats, fiber, and iron, so give them a try.

Ezekiel Bread Avocado Toast
Next on the list is a lower-calorie twist on a popular dish consumed nearly everywhere. Avocado toast is already a pretty

filling meal on its own but can be somewhat inconsistent from a calorie density perspective. Depending on the type of bread used, a slice of avocado toast can range anywhere from 180-300 calories, so fitting it into a weight loss plan could be tricky. Luckily, there is a solution, and its name is Ezekiel. A slice of Ezekiel bread ranks high on the satiety index and low in calories, meaning you can enjoy a fair bit of it before the Kcals (kilocalories) start adding up. Avocados are also very filling and contain many antioxidants and vitamin C, so you can never go wrong with them. If your lifestyle allows it, you can also add an egg to the dish to round out the satiety and add a little protein to the mix.

Hummus and Baby Carrots
Hummus and carrots make for excellent snacks to pull out of your fridge when feeling peckish. Both foods are low-calories and will fill you up quickly, making them ideal replacements for standard calorie-dense options like potato chips or sugary candies. If you want to add a little zest to the dish, you can always drizzle a bit of lemon juice and a pinch of salt to add that extra bit of flavor you might be craving. Like most food items on this list, hummus and carrots are chock-full of essential vitamins, including calcium, vitamin A, and potassium. Best of all, hummus and carrots are dirt cheap and contain a lot of fiber to lower cholesterol levels and regulate healthy bowel movements.

Lentil Soup
The last dish on the list is filling, low in calories, and perfect for keeping warm during those cold winter nights. Lentil soup is a typical dish found in many cultures worldwide, so finding the necessary ingredients is simple. There is also a wealth of different recipes and prep methods available online, allowing you to continue to make enjoyable new combinations. Like other meals on this list, lentil soup contains a healthy serving of protein, carbohydrates, and essential micronutrients, including B vitamins, magnesium, and zinc. Lentils, like most vegetables, rank very high in satiety, and the addition of broth will have you feel-

ing satisfied in no time.

The four meals mentioned above are affordable, nutrient-dense, low in calories, and most importantly, accessible to all dietary lifestyles (i.e., vegan, vegetarian, etc.). They are also easy to experiment with by adding other ingredients and trying different preparations, leaving you a lot of room to get truly creative. If you are looking to spice things up in the kitchen and achieve your weight loss milestones with a more enjoyable lifestyle approach to dieting, then these four options are sure to do the trick.

TIP #7: MAKE WATER PART OF YOUR WEIGHT-LOSS PLAN

Water plays a crucial role in human health. This is not surprising, considering that the human body is 60 percent water. When you are dehydrated, your body does not function efficiently. And this adversely affects functions that range from burning body fat to critical thinking.

On weight loss, research suggests that being adequately hydrated can make your workouts more efficient and boost your metabolism - that is, the way your body converts food into energy. Drinking water before eating could also suppress your appetite. Below are ways water aids in weight loss.

- **It makes your workouts more efficient**

Your body needs water during exercise. According to dietitians, water dissolves magnesium, sodium and potassium, and transports the minerals throughout the body. The electrical energy produced triggers muscle contractions needed for movement.

When you exercise with too little water in your body, you risk developing cramps. In addition, dehydrated cells build muscle more slowly than hydrated cells, making your workouts less efficient. Being hydrated adequately can decrease fatigue, meaning you can exercise for longer and burn more calories. It's best to hydrate before and during exercise. In addition, according to a 2016 mini-review published in Frontiers in Nutrition, adequate hydration may increase your body's ability to burn fat.

- **It boosts your metabolism**

Studies suggest that adequate hydration fuels your body's metabolism, leading to weight loss. In a 2013 study by researchers associated with Pad Dr D Y Patil Medical College and Hospital, Nerul, in Navi Mumbai, India, 50 overweight girls drank two cups of water 30 minutes before breakfast, lunch and dinner. They made no additional dietary changes. After eight weeks, the girls lost weight and recorded a reduction in body mass index and body composition scores.

According to dietitians, when you drink cold water, your body has to use energy to warm the water to body temperature. This produces heat, and the more energy your body uses, the faster your metabolism.

In a small 2003 study, when 14 healthy adults drank 500 ml of 71° F (21.6° C) water, their metabolism rate increased by 30 percent on average. The increase happened within 10 minutes, peaking after 30 to 40 minutes. The study was published in the Journal of Clinical Endocrinology & Metabolism.

- **Water may suppress your appetite**

Drinking water before your meal helps to make you feel full, thus reducing the amount of food you eat. In a small 2016 study, 14 young males who drank about 500 ml of water just before a meal ended up eating 22 percent less than those who didn't take water. The researchers, led by Robert A Corney of the School of Sport, Exercise and Health Sciences, Loughborough University, Loughborough, Leicestershire, UK, suggested drinking water before a meal could aid in weight loss.

Again, sometimes you may mistake thirst for hunger. Nutritionists suggest you first look for water when you think you're hungry. You may find you are thirsty instead and only need water.

- **Proper hydration may boost alertness**

Water may boost alertness. Dehydration may cause drowsiness and reduced alertness, according to researchers of the 2016 mini-review. When you are dehydrated, you may suffer bouts of dizziness and fatigue and become de-motivated to exercise, and may make unhealthy food choices. Research suggests that your brain, just like your body, needs water to function optimally. Dehydration weakens your brain's ability to perform cognitive, memory and physical functions.

Final thoughts

Replace juice, soda, alcohol and other high-calorie drinks with water. This will cut down on your calorie intake. Drinking water may not come easily to everyone. You may be willing to drink water just when you're thirsty. To get around this limitation, adopt the habit of drinking water throughout the day, sipping it all day. Make drinking water part of your normal routine.

Secondly, it's best to drink water half an hour before eating and again half an hour after eating. Drinking water with your meal could dilute the digestive gastric juice, making digestion difficult. If you are very thirsty and must drink water with your food, take a few sips. Don't down a whole glass.

As for weight loss, water is not a magic bullet that will get rid of the excess weight. You also need to make healthy food choices, watch your food portions, and keep physically active.

PART B: EXERCISE TIPS

In this section, you'll find out the benefits of making exercise a part of your weekly routine. Exercise offers truly life-changing results if you're willing to put in the effort required. A lean or muscular body is an obvious benefit, but does exercising offer anything else? The answer is yes.

TIP #8: FOODS TO EAT BEFORE AND AFTER RUNNING

Nothing feels better than a good, long run with the wind in your hair and the sounds of the city or country. Without a doubt, long runs will burn a great deal of energy. This means it is very important for runners to eat, both before and after their runs. Before a run, food needs to be consumed 30 to 60 minutes earlier. After a run, it is best to feed your muscles within 30 minutes.

Foods to Eat Before the Run
First and foremost, before eating any food at all, it is best for runners to drink water. It is important to hydrate yourself with 12 to 16 ounces of water roughly an hour prior to your workout. Bringing water along with you on your run is also a great idea.

The best thing to eat prior to your run is something loaded with carbohydrates balanced with proteins. This will help you burn fat during your workout. It is also best to eat foods that are easy to digest, such as those low in fat and fiber.

If you are going on a short run, under an hour, some snacks you can eat prior to your workout include:
- Half a Clif bar or other power bar
- Fruit, such as a banana or peach
- An English muffin with jelly or jam
- Applesauce or pudding

If you are going on a longer run, over an hour, some snacks you can eat prior to your workout include:
- A cup of Greek yogurt

- A banana with peanut or almond butter
- 2 slices of wholewheat bread with peanut or almond butter
- 1 cooked sweet potato
- Cooked oatmeal or quinoa
- Hummus

In order to avoid cramps while running, it is important not to eat too much. Eating until you are satisfied rather than full will help. Make sure you eat at least 30 minutes before your workout to stay pain-free.

Foods to Eat After the Run

After a run, it is important to replenish energy as soon as possible. Muscles are ready for their refuel within 30 minutes of the run. They are very receptive to restoring glycogen immediately after you run. In the long run, eating right after running will also help you reduce muscle soreness and stiffness. Eating a large amount of carbohydrates after the run is just as important as eating them beforehand. After a long workout, you need to make sure you are feeding your body so it can continue to burn fat and also replenish itself of all the vitamins and minerals consumed.

For those able to stomach food immediately after a run, some post-run food options include:
- A bagel with peanut butter
- A fruit and yogurt smoothie
- A Clif or other protein bar
- Hummus
- Chicken breast
- Salmon
- Almonds

If you are not able to quite stomach food after a long run, drinking chocolate milk is a good option. The milk provides B vitamins and carbohydrates, making it a good drink for recovery.

Drinking plenty of water to rehydrate the body is also important after a long run.

Why Carbohydrates?
As you have likely noticed, the best foods to consume before and after a run are carbohydrates. The same principles can be applied to other strenuous workouts. The nutrients are important for athletes of all calibers to maximize speed, energy levels, focus, endurance, and fluid balance. Basically, they are the body's fuel.

Carbohydrates, in the form of muscle glycogen, play a particularly major role in an athlete's body because they also enable your body's protein to be used for tissue synthesis or muscle building. It helps you build endurance and allows you to work out at an intense level.

TIP #9: HOW JOGGING AFFECTS YOUR BODY

There's no specific timetable for seeing positive changes in your body after you've taken up jogging. The benefits of jogging begin immediately and tend to increase over time; you'll see even more marked improvement at a year and six months.

Weight-Loss

Whether you lose weight and how much weight you lose depends upon several factors, including how much time you spend jogging and how much food you eat every day. Harvard Health Publications reports that a 155-pound person will burn about 230 calories in 30 minutes doing a light jog/walk. You'll have to burn 3,500 calories for every pound of weight you want to lose, but after a month or so, you should be seeing some weight-loss.

Muscle Development

In your first few days of jogging, you likely felt sore after a jog. This phenomenon, called delayed-onset muscle soreness, is a product of tiny tears in your muscles. These tears help build new, healthy muscle tissue, and DOMS tends to decrease with regular exercise. After a few weeks, you might feel a little sore after a jog, but severe soreness should reduce. You might also notice more muscle development both because you're shedding fat and building muscle in your legs.

Physical Health

Regular jogging can improve your cardiovascular health by strengthening your cardiac muscle and improving circulation. Over time, you may see a drop in blood pressure and lower pulse.

Over time you may notice that you feel less breathless after jogging, and your heart rate might drop slightly. Jogging also strengthens your lungs, enabling them to work more effectively with your heart, and you may notice you have a higher lung capacity.

Mental Health
The benefits of jogging do not end with your body. You may also notice an improvement in your mood. During a heavy jog, your body releases endorphins that can give you a temporary feel-good rush. Over time, though, jogging can improve your mood on a longer term basis and make it easier to get quality sleep. According to the U.S. Centers for Disease Control and Prevention, you'll need 30 to 60 minutes of physical activity every day to reduce your risk of depression and see an improvement in sleep.

TIP #10: WALKING, JOGGING, OR RUNNING - WHAT'S BEST FOR YOUR HEALTH?

Walking, jogging, and running are all cardiovascular activities. They increase the heartbeat and breathing. You might be at a loss as to what to choose to keep fit. All three exercises can help you control your weight and improve your heart and mental health.

So, which should you choose? Let's look at some considerations to help you decide.

- **Injury and damage to joints**

Running and jogging can damage your joints, but walking is gentler on your joints, particularly the knees. Walking also reduces the risk of injury. When walking, you move your body-weight gently from one foot to the other compared to when running or jogging, you push all your body weight on to one foot with force as you land on the ground.

A study by researchers affiliated to the Division of Cancer Prevention at the National Institutes of Health at Bethesda, Maryland, USA, concluded that the risk of injury in young men who run or jog is 25 percent higher than for those who walk. The study, published in the Clinical Journal of Sports Medicine, further established that when you run, you exert pressure on your joints that's 2.5 times your body weight. Walking, in comparison, uses a force 1.2 times your body weight. Overall, more than 50 percent of runners suffer some injury, whereas only about 1 percent of walkers are injured. Moreover, you're more likely to trip and fall when running than when walking.

• **Longevity**

A study by researchers associated with the Department of Public Health of Japan's Hokkaido University concluded that regular walking might improve longevity in elderly men. The study, published in 2015, indicated that the findings apply regardless of the men's lifestyle, medical status, or body mass index (BMI).

Jogging too, carries longevity benefits. An investigation, Longevity in Male and Female Joggers: The Copenhagen City Heart Study, connected both male and female joggers to longer lives than non-joggers. The study was published in the American Journal of Epidemiology of April 1, 2013.

• **Heart rate and heart disease**

When you jog or run, your heart rate rises to around 120-130 beats a minute. Walking does its bit too. When you walk at a brisk rate of about 100 steps per minute, you raise your heartbeat to about 100 beats per minute. Therefore, running, jogging, and walking all improve your fitness level.

Nevertheless, there's a caution about running. In an observational study that tracked over 52,000 people for 30 years, researchers found that the death risk for runners was 19 percent lower than that of non-runners. However, the benefits declined for those who ran faster than eight miles an hour or further than 20 miles a week. This is certainly not a case of the more the better.

According to this study published in Medicine and Science in Sports & Exercise, runners benefited if they ran 19 miles a week at six to seven miles an hour. More than this and the risk of death equaled that of sedentary people.

There's more. Research from Lawrence Berkeley National

Laboratory, USA, found that heart disease went down by 9.3 percent in walkers, but by only 4.5 percent in runners. In addition, risks for first-time hypertension and high cholesterol were lowered more by walking than running.

- **Weight loss**

Joggers and runners lose more weight faster, than walkers do. A study by Human Performance Laboratory, Appalachian State University, North Carolina Research Campus, Kannapolis, USA, concluded that vigorous activity increases metabolic rate and burns more calories than less intense exercise. You thus lose more weight per hour of exercise when running and jogging than when walking. However, you need to consider the other factors mentioned here.

Bottom line

Running and jogging deliver more benefits per hour of work than walking. However, you need to take into account the risks of injury that running and jogging present. Also, ask yourself if you're able to sustain a running and jogging regimen to meet the World Health Organization (WHO) recommendations for health. For adults aged 18 to 64 years, WHO recommends at least 150 minutes of moderate-intensity aerobic activity spread over the week, or at least 75 minutes of vigorous-intensity aerobic exercises. Alternatively, you could engage in an equivalent mixture of a moderate and vigorous-intensity workout.

The decision is yours, depending on your health, age, weight, and interest. If you are ready, you could run or jog for say, two days a week, and walk on the other days.

TIP #11: WHY YOU NEED TO DO ANAEROBIC EXERCISES IN CONJUNCTION WITH AEROBICS

Everybody knows that you need to get plenty of exercise on a regular basis. However, the type of exercise you are doing is every bit as important as the amount of time you spend exercising. Doing equal amounts of aerobic exercises and anaerobic exercises is the best way to get the complete workout that you need.

The Difference between Aerobic and Anaerobic Exercise
Exercise comes in two categories: aerobic and anaerobic. There are three primary differences between them: the way your muscles contract, the number of reps you do in a set, and the way your muscles generate energy.

Aerobic exercises involve low to moderate amount of resistance, so your muscles contract quickly and easily. Because of this, you can do a lot of reps per set. During aerobic exercise, your muscles get their energy from breaking down glycogen, which is an energy-dense sugar that your body uses to store energy, by using oxygen. At a moderate level of exercise intensity, your muscles can rely on this process for long periods of time. Aerobic exercises include such activities as jogging, cycling, and swimming.

Anaerobic exercise uses high levels of resistance, so your muscles really need to work in order to contract. Because of this, you can only do a few reps per set. During anaerobic exercise, the demand placed on your muscles requires more oxygen than your body has available, so the aerobic method of energy production becomes impossible. To counteract this, your body starts breaking down glycogen using other means than oxygen in a process called glycolysis. This process creates a lot of lactic acid in your muscles, which is what makes them feel like they burn after a short period of exercise. Anaerobic exercises are done in short bursts, and include weight lifting, High Intensity Interval Training (or HIIT), and sprinting.

The Benefits of Aerobic Exercise

You build up your endurance with aerobic exercises, allowing you to do everything you do for longer before you get tired. Aerobic exercise also improves your cardiovascular fitness, which lowers your heart rate and blood pressure, even when you're not exercising. It also helps you lose weight and boosts your immune system.

The Benefits of Anaerobic Exercise

You build up your strength with anaerobic exercises. Anaerobic exercises also help you lose weight, but they do it even better than aerobic exercises do. They help increase your bone density, making you more resistant to fractures and to osteoporosis. The strength gains you get from aerobic exercises can also protect your joints.

Medical Concerns

If you have any health problems, or if you don't know how to put together a safe, effective workout incorporating both aerobic and anaerobic exercise, you should check with your doctor. Your doctor can help you develop an exercise routine that ensures you safely get enough of both types of exercise.

Final Thoughts

Even the strongest bodybuilder will not be able to get a lot of use out of their strength without the endurance that aerobics develop, and no matter how long you swim or jog, you'll never improve your strength or burn fat with much effectiveness. If you want to be truly healthy then you need both aerobic and anaerobic exercises.

TIP #12: HOW TO GET YOUR MOTIVATION BACK AND HIT THOSE FITNESS GOALS

Remember how it was right after you decided to start exercising and get in shape? It was easy to do it in the early days. You had a lot of energy, enthusiasm, and resolution. But as time went by, your motivation to exercise got weaker and weaker. And now, you frequently don't work out at all, and when you do, you don't bring your A-game. You know you need to get your motivation back, but not how to get it back. Fortunately, there are things you can do that can help.

Start Cross-Training

The most common de-motivator is, perhaps, boredom. If you've been doing the same routine forever, you may simply need a change. So swap out some or all of the exercises you do now with different ones. Replace jogging with swimming, perhaps. Use different lifts than you usually use. The specifics don't much matter so long as your routine is new. Also, by cross-training, you'll work out more muscles, including the ones your usual routine misses. You'll get more fit as a result.

Review Your Goals

Your lack of motivation might be a problem with your goals. If your exercise goals are too easy to meet, you'll get bored with your workouts. If your goals are too difficult to meet, you'll get discouraged and start feeling like it's pointless to even try. If you're not feeling the desire to exercise, take a good look at your exercise goals. Be honest with yourself. Are they realistic? Are they too easy? If you answer yes to either question, you need to set new goals.

Review the Way You Reward Yourself

A lot of people motivate themselves to exercise by rewarding themselves when they do, and there's nothing wrong with that. Unless, of course, you're going too far with your rewards. If you aren't making any progress toward your fitness or weight-loss goals, the discouragement you feel could be causing your lack of motivation. Take an honest look at the way you reward yourself. On days you exercise, do you let yourself eat a lot of junk food? Do you, other than the exercise, let yourself be more sedentary than normal? You could be sabotaging your own efforts by rewarding yourself with counterproductive treats.

Stay Away From the Scale

If you are exercising to lose weight, you're probably checking the scale a lot to see how you're doing. If you're not making progress fast enough, that could be discouraging you. If you feel stressed out about your lack of weight-loss progress, stay away from the scale for a while. Just work out and don't get too hung up on the results. If you can let go of the worry, you might find that working out is more fun.

Final Thoughts

There's a good reason why you're not feeling motivated to work out. If you find that reason, you can do something about it. Fitness is as much about mental factors as it is about physical ones.

PART C: HEALTHY EATING TIPS

The delicious aroma and taste of food draws us to eating it. In this section, your perception about diet will change and you'll also be introduced to delicious foods with several health benefits along with tips to distance yourself from unhealthy food.

TIP #13: CLEAN EATING IS EASIER THAN YOU MAY THINK

You've probably heard that clean eating has significant health benefits. But for those not familiar with the particulars of clean eating, it can seem overwhelming. Many believe it's an expensive and difficult change of habit. The truth is it's less complicated and more affordable than you may think.

One misconception that can turn people off is that clean eating is too complicated. Like any lifestyle change, it takes some initial effort. However, it is not complicated. The effort comes from changing the way you look at food and getting used to cooking whole meals instead of using boxes and jars.

The easiest way to begin is by making a few food swaps. What you're trying to achieve is replacing processed food with whole, natural food. Evaluate any processed food you have in your kitchen. These may include frozen meals, boxed pasta meals, and jars and packets of sauces. These have many ingredients that you don't need and can damage your health. These include added fat, sugar, sodium, chemicals, and preservatives. Imagine what whole ingredients you can put together to achieve the same flavor profiles you find in processed food. The flavors you can create with a few whole ingredients and little time may surprise you.

Start by leaving boxed pasta and rice meals on the store shelves. Cook plain pasta and rice with raw vegetables, spices, and herbs. Make your own spice mixes instead of using ready-made packets. Use plain oats. Add fresh fruit, pure honey, and cinnamon. Ditch the chemically processed vegetable and canola oils, as well as margarine. Opt for cold-pressed coconut and olive oils that are high in quality. Replace flavored yogurt with plain yogurt and mix in fresh fruit. Instead of drinking fruit juices loaded with sugar, eat whole pieces of fruit. Then, enjoy a crisp glass of water or a cup of tea. Processed meat is another food you'll want to avoid. Choose grass fed meats that are free of hormones and antibiotics. Search for clean marinara sauce recipes. You'll find most are simple, timely, and much better than the jarred stuff.

Once you've decided on swaps, you'll need to approach shopping a little differently than usual. At the grocery store, read labels on everything you buy. Make sure packaged, canned, and frozen foods have few ingredients. Long lists of ingredients that you have trouble understanding are red flags. Aside from unpronounceable chemicals and preservatives, beware of trans fats, salt, and sugar.

Expense is also a concern for many people while shopping for healthy food. The general belief that clean eating is expensive has some foundation. Past studies have shown that processed food costs less per calorie than whole foods cost. But that's not the whole story here. Processed food can have negative impacts on your health. Over time, disease prevention and treatment can cost more than eating healthy food. Also, other studies have shown a decreasing gap in price points with rising demand for nutritious food. Affording healthy food is also a matter of arming yourself with information that allows you to shop and eat smart.

One of the most obvious ways to save money on groceries is also one of the simplest ways: buy in-season produce. Two major factors make produce more expensive when out of season than when in season. The first is the excess cost of shipping from a place in which the produce is in season. The second is the high energy cost of forcing growth of produce that is out of season.

Local growers must replicate natural environments to bring this produce into stores.

Because of these reasons, you're always going to save on in-season produce. During fall and winter, pick root vegetables. Choose greens such as Brussels sprouts, collards, and cabbage. Buy apples, oranges, grapefruits, and pears. In spring and summer, pick vegetables such as corn, eggplant, asparagus, bell peppers, and tomatoes. Stick with fruits like nectarines, watermelon, apricots, plums, and strawberries. Apples are typically in season all year, though they tend to be least expensive during the fall. Many fruits and vegetables also overlap seasons, so look out for price trends.

The next way to save money while eating well is to buy certain items in bulk. Dry beans, rice, lentils, barley, and quinoa are great options for buying in bulk. They're often cheaper per unit of weight than small packages. Look at the price labels on the shelves of everything you buy. Compare the prices per unit of measure on bulk and non-bulk packages to determine the best buy.

Another way to stock up and save money is by buying canned and frozen fruits, vegetables, and beans. Look for varieties of vegetables and beans that advertise no added salt. Buy fruit in natural juices (not syrup). Try the store brand of these items, and watch for sales. This also reduces the waste that happens when produce goes rancid faster than you can use it.

Now that you have a pantry and refrigerator full of healthy food, make preparing your meals fun. Play around, and find what you love. You don't have to be a superstar chef to create delicious meals with whole ingredients. Experiment with different flavor combinations, and think of it as healthful creation instead of a chore.

Clean eating does not have to be overwhelming. It's easier than you may think to nourish your body with healthy food choices. Commit to informing yourself, cooking with whole foods, and shopping smart to stick within your budget.

TIP #14: SEVEN IRON-RICH FOODS TO BOOST YOUR ENERGY LEVELS

Iron deficiency is one of the most common causes of chronic tiredness and fatigue. Inadequate iron intake can lead to iron-deficiency anaemia, which causes tiredness, shortness of breath and pale skin. Iron supplements can have unpleasant side effects, such as constipation and stomach pain, which means that many people prefer to boost their iron intake by increasing the amount of iron in their diet. Here are 7 iron-rich foods to boost your energy levels.

Liver

Liver is one of the best foods to eat if you are anaemic, as it contains high amounts of iron. Liver also contains vitamins A, C, D and E, which are essential for the human body to function properly. In addition, liver provides a wealth of other important nutrients, including phosphorous, calcium, magnesium, zinc, potassium and copper. Chicken liver, beef liver and lambs liver are all excellent sources of iron and can be cooked in a variety of dishes.

Red Meat

Red meat is another excellent source of iron, with 100 grams of red meat containing around 3 milligrams of iron, depending on the type of meat and method of cooking. Red meat also contains vitamins A, C, B6 and B12, as well as calcium, magnesium, potassium and folic acid. If you are worried about the high fat content of some red meats, choose lean cuts or thin steaks, remembering to trim any visible fat from the meat.

Eggs

Eggs are high in protein and full of essential nutrients, including vitamin A, vitamin D, vitamin E, vitamin K, calcium, zinc, phosphorous and selenium. Eggs also contain high quantities of iron, with two large eggs giving you around 1 milligram of iron. Many of the nutrients found in eggs are contained in the yolk, so you will need to eat the whole egg to gain maximum benefits.

Dried Fruit

Dried fruit contains high amounts of iron. Dried apricots, in particular, can give you a substantial iron boost. In addition, dried apricots contain significant amounts of vitamin A and vitamin C, as well as dietary fiber, which is essential for a healthy digestive system. Prunes and raisins also contain generous amounts of iron and other nutrients.

Leafy Greens

Leafy green vegetables are packed with healthy nutrients, including iron, calcium, magnesium and a whole range of vitamins. Spinach is one of the best vegetable sources of iron, particularly when eaten raw. Vegans may find it difficult to obtain adequate amounts of iron from their diet, as the best food sources of iron come from animal products, so it is important for vegans to eat plenty of leafy green vegetables.

Dark Chocolate

Dark chocolate can contain around 17 milligrams of iron per 100 grams of chocolate, depending on the amount of cocoa it contains. Milk chocolate does not contain the same nutritional benefits, as it contains less cocoa powder. Cocoa powder contains high amounts of iron and can be found in dark chocolate and cocoa-based drinks. Dark chocolate also contains powerful antioxidants that help to reduce harmful pollutants in the body.

Fortified Breakfast Cereals

Many breakfast cereals are now fortified with iron and other nutrients. Check the label to see which vitamins, minerals and nutrients have been added to your cereal. While fortified cereals can help to boost your iron intake, many of these cereals contain high amounts of sugar and salt, so it is important to keep an eye on the labels when buying breakfast cereal.

Eating plenty of iron in your diet can help to boost your energy levels and reduce the risk of developing anaemia. In order to absorb iron effectively, your body needs an adequate supply of vitamin C. Vitamin C can be found in oranges, strawberries, red peppers, broccoli and potatoes.

TIP #15: THESE 7 FRUITS AND VEGETABLES ARE THE MOST LIKELY TO CAUSE BLOATING

Bloating is that uncomfortable feeling of fullness in the middle of your tummy. If you have a lot of bloating, your abdomen may be visually distended, and it may be hard to zip up your pants. It's not uncommon to develop a little bloating after eating a heavy meal, especially if you eat too quickly, but some people have it frequently and when they eat certain foods.

As you might expect, bloating is often caused by diet, including food intolerances, and some of the healthiest foods can cause it. When confronted with bloating, most people focus on the obvious culprits -- foods containing gluten and dairy. But many vegetables can expand your tummy with gas and make you feel uncomfortable. Let's look at the most common culprits for bloating in the produce department.

1. Broccoli
There are few vegetables that are healthier than broccoli, a cruciferous vegetable linked with anti-inflammatory activity. Scientists also point out that broccoli contains compounds called glucosinolates that your body converts to sulforaphane. Some laboratory studies show that sulforaphane slows the growth of certain cancers.

The downside to broccoli is it can cause bloating, especially if you eat it raw or eat too much before your intestinal tract has a chance to adapt. Broccoli contains a sugar called raffinose that your digestive tract can't break down. But when gut bacteria get a hold of raffinose, they ferment and turn it into gases that cause bloating.

2. Kale

Kale is another cruciferous vegetable that has similar benefits and problems that broccoli does. This green, leafy vegetable contains the sugar raffinose that bacteria feed on and convert to waistline-expanding gas. If you love kale but it causes bloating and gas, you still have a recourse. According to dietitians, marinating kale in lemon juice for 8 hours breaks down the raffinose that causes you to bloat. The lemon also provides extra vitamin C too.

3. Cabbage

Add cabbage to the list of cruciferous vegetables that contain raffinose. Although cabbage is rich in vitamins, minerals, and phytonutrients, it can be a belly expander if you eat too much of it. So, eat it in smaller amounts and cook it beforehand. Bonus points for buying red cabbage; it contains purple pigments called anthocyanins with anti-inflammatory activity.

4. Onions

Onions are another gas-forming vegetable, but not for the same reasons as broccoli, kale, and cabbage. Onions contain fructans, a type of fiber that triggers bloating in some people. People vary in their susceptibility to fructans, but you'll also find them in other foods, including garlic, wheat, and leeks. It doesn't take much onion to cause bloating either. One way to reduce bloating from onions is to cook them before placing them on your plate.

5. Apples

Apples are one of the healthiest fruits there is, and also high in fiber. However, apples contain a copious amount of a sugar called fructose that some people have a hard time breaking down, but bacteria love it and produce gas when they munch on it. They also contain a sugar alcohol called sorbitol that can cause bloating. Still, apples are a nutritious snack and are better for you than any type of processed snack you can buy.

6. Pears

Yep! Pears contain fructose too, which makes them a fruit likely to cause bloating, along with apples. Of the two fructose-rich fruits, apples have a slight nutritional advantage. They contain a variety of vitamins and minerals, and several key phytonutrients, like quercetin, with anti-inflammatory activity. Overall, they're a bit more nutritious than pears. Plus, more studies have looked at the health properties of apples than pears. For example, a 2011 study linked a diet rich in apples with lower rates of a number of cancers, including cancer of the prostate, breast, ovary, colon, oral cavity, and esophagus.

7. Beans

Beans aren't exactly a vegetable, but they are a plant-based food that causes bloating. The reason? Beans contain carbohydrates called oligosaccharides that your digestive tract has a hard time breaking down. To break down the oligosaccharides in beans, you need an enzyme called alpha-galactosidase that your body can't make. On the plus side, you can get this enzyme from an over-the-counter product called Beano sold at many pharmacies. Bean lovers pop a Beano before eating beans to reduce their gas-forming tendency.

Another trick: Soaking beans overnight in water and discarding the water before cooking will reduce their ability to form gas. Another tip is to cook beans with kombu, type of dried seaweed. Kombu contains the alpha-galactosidase enzyme you need to break down oligosaccharides in beans.

The Bottom Line

Now you have the lowdown on the fruits and vegetables likely to cause gas, and can adjust your diet accordingly. If you have persistent bloating despite making dietary changes, consult your healthcare provider. There are also medical causes of bloating, some of which are serious.

TIP #16: YOUR HEALTHY GROCERY LIST – TIPS FOR HEALTHY SUPERMARKET SHOPPING

Eating healthy is important, but you cannot whip up a healthy meal if there is no food in the house. Your healthy eating habits start where you buy your food - at the local grocery store or supermarket.

You do not have to blow your entire paycheck at the organic grocery or health food store. With a little bit of planning and some old fashioned discipline, you can find great healthy ingredients at your regular store. Just use these simple tips to get started.

- **Check the list of ingredients** - the size of the ingredient list matters a lot. If that ingredient list takes up half the package, chances are the product is heavily processed and potentially unhealthy.

- **Read the label** - the nutritional label is full of useful information, from the number of calories per serving to the amount of fat and the fiber content. Get in the habit of reading those labels, and use that information to make smart buying decisions.

- **Start with the produce section** - fill your shopping cart in the produce section, focusing on healthy in season fruits and vegetables. Fruits and vegetables should make up a large portion of every meal. Make sure they represent a large portion of your shopping basket as well.

- Shop the perimeter of the store - the outer sections of the grocery store are often home to the healthiest choices. From produce to fresh cut meats and healthy seafood, the perimeter of the store is a great place to find healthy food.

- Look for fresh herbs and spices - those dried and bottled spices are fine in a pinch, but fresh is always better. Look for fresh garlic bulbs and grind your own for those great recipes. Buy fresh basil and dry it for long-term storage. Fresh herbs taste better, and they are better for you as well.

- Use sales to stock up on healthy staples - it is a sad reality that healthy items are often more expensive than junk food. Fight back by stocking up on those healthy staples when they go on sale. Watch the weekly circulars, make your list and buy in bulk to save money.

- Get to know your local butcher - the butcher at your grocery store can be your best ally in your quest for healthy cooking. Ask your new best friend to trim the fat from those roasts and steaks before you buy them, or to choose the leanest cuts of meat for your family.

- Choose whole grain breads and pastas - switching from heavily processed white bread and bleached pasta to whole grain varieties is one of the best things you can do for your health.

- Watch out for products marketed to kids - even if you have children, it pays to stay away from cereals, juices and other products that are targeted at them. These products often contain lots of added sugars and other potentially harmful ingredients.

- Watch those percentages - when shopping for juice, look for 100% juice on the label. Many seemingly healthy juices are loaded down with added sugars and artificial ingredients.

TIP #17: INCREDIBLE HEALTH BENEFITS OF A RAW FOOD DIET

With so many different diet and exercise plans on the market, it can be hard to know what you should be doing to improve your physical condition. Should you try one of the extreme diets that make you lose weight by almost starving yourself? Do you incorporate an extensive and exhausting exercise regime into your life?

What if you could lose weight and balance your health needs by simply changing what you eat. Rather than ticking off lists of foods you can't have, why not think outside the box? The main problem with most weight loss diets is that they are not sustainable. You will eventually do yourself more damage by cutting off essential nutrients in various types of food. However, a popular dietary option is the raw food diet, and although it can be discouraging in the beginning, it can be a sustainable dietary choice.

While on a raw food diet, you eat only raw food, but this does not limit you to what you can eat. This means you can still eat fish, fruit, vegetables, meat, and dairy. You can eat anything as long as it is raw. The bonus of a raw diet is that it produces enzymes in your body which helps increase metabolism, aiding weight loss in the process. Not only does this make your job to watch your overall health easier, but it will also aid in making you healthier for longer.

Not only that, but it can be a genuine long-term dietary plan. While being the hardest part, once you are used to eating only raw products, then you will start to see positive physical results. It makes serving food quick and easy, cutting down on hunger pains and gives you an easy, long-term option when it comes to the food you eat. It may take a little time to get used to at the start, but once the positive health benefits start to show, you will find it easier to continue on.

Raw foods are also reported to give you more energy than when cooked. This is believed to be related to eating less fat and grease. Even so, most people on a raw food diet agree that since starting to eat only raw foods, they feel more active and ready to go at the start of each day. Raw food diets can also be beneficial in reducing the amount of cholesterol your body consumes and in turn, can help maintain a healthier heart.

One of the main benefits to a diet of this type, however, is that it can help you feel better physically and mentally. Not only will you feel better inside, but cutting back on all the fatty excesses you were eating previously will help clear your skin as well due to the huge quantities of antioxidants in raw fruit and vegetables. So not only will you feel better, you will look healthier too.

Although it can be difficult to get started, once you get past the first few weeks, you should find a raw food diet to be extremely beneficial for your weight loss goals and overall health. The hardest part for many people is adjusting to the taste, but if you push through and continue on, you will be able to see the many incredible health benefits for yourself.

TIP #18: TEN WAYS TO REDUCE UNHEALTHY FAT IN YOUR DAILY DIET

If you want to live a healthier lifestyle, reducing the fat in your daily diet is a great place to start. Many of us are consuming more fat than we even realize. That hidden fat can really add up, resulting in extra pounds and even chronic health problems.

You can use these tips to cut the amount of fat in your diet and get on the road to a healthier and happier lifestyle.

- **Swap out full fat milk for skim or reduced fat versions.** Regular milk is high in fat and calories. Simply switching to skim and reduced fat milk can help you lose weight and reduce your daily fat intake.

- **Swap out regular ice cream and enjoy non-fat frozen yogurt instead.** Frozen yogurt comes in an amazing variety of flavors, nearly as many as regular ice cream. You do not have to give up variety or good taste to reduce fat and calories.

- **Choose the leanest ground beef you can find.** Ground beef is rated on its fat content, i.e. 85% lean and 15% fat. Always choose the lowest fat ground beef you can find.

- **Switch to low fat ground turkey instead.** You can reduce fat even more by switching to ground turkey for your hamburgers and your favorite recipes. Ground turkey is delicious - and much lower in fat than most ground beef.

- **Trim the fat off your steaks before they hit the grill.** Trimming the visible fat off your steaks can make them healthier for you. If you prefer to cook your steaks with the fat on, be sure to trim the fat when they hit the table.

- **Reduce the amount of sauces, gravies and dressings you use in your cooking and on your food.** Don't ruin that healthy salad by loading it up with fatty blue cheese or ranch dressing. Go easy on the sauces when you cook, and avoid the temptation to pile them on at the table.

-**Watch out for hidden fats in baked goods**. That healthy looking muffin could be harboring lots of saturated fat. You can control the amount of fat in those sweet treats by making your own cookies, cakes and pies. Choosing low fat ingredients can allow you to indulge your sweet tooth in a healthy way.

- **Avoid fried foods whenever you can.** Use healthy cooking techniques like broiling, baking and grilling when you cook at home. Cooking healthy is a great way to reduce the fat in your daily diet.

- **Remove the skin from chicken and turkey before you eat.** That skin is full of fat, and it soaks up additional grease and fat during cooking. If you cooked the poultry properly, removing the skin should not affect moisture or flavor.

- **Check the nutrition information on the menu when you eat out.** Restaurant meals are notorious for hidden fat. Check the fat content before you order, and ask your server if the dish can be prepared in a more healthy manner.

TIP #19: THREE WAYS TO GET YOUR MORNING BOOST

Most of us aren't naturally morning people. We might take a few minutes to roll out of bed and stumble into the bathroom to prepare for our day. One of the best things about the weekend is that we're not on a schedule – there's no set time we have to wake up and get moving. For the typical nine-to-five worker, however, every weekday begins with a grumpy, drowsy, and unfocused hour. The ultimate necessity of going to work is the only factor motivating many people to make it out of their front doors before 10 AM.

If you find yourself wishing that you could just call in sick and crawl back into bed, you might need an extra boost to properly kick off your day. Try changing your early morning diet in the following ways.

1) Eat a real breakfast.
Many of us, desiring the maximum amount of sleep possible before the workday begins, put off getting up to the last minute. As a result, our only breakfast is a cup of coffee and one of those little breakfast cereal bars that seem to be lighter than air and don't fill us at all. This is undoubtedly a fast breakfast; it can even be consumed in the car or on the train on the way to work. However, it is not the most efficient breakfast possible.

As inconvenient as it might seem, try waking up early enough to give yourself the time to make a real breakfast before work. A good weekday breakfast should be light and include a mix of carbohydrates and protein. Eggs and toast only take a few minutes to prepare, and they make a classic breakfast for good reason – the protein in the eggs and the carbohydrates in the bread will give you the base of energy necessary to take on the rest of the day, or at least up until you get a break for lunch.

2) Include nuts and citrus in your weekday breakfast.

Nuts and fruits are not usually regarded as typical breakfast foods. Fruits tend to be left over for the much heavier weekend breakfast, while nuts are often ignored altogether. However, including a handful of almonds or an orange in your weekday breakfast can give you a much-needed extra boost of energy. Many nuts, such as almonds, cashews, and hazelnuts, are convenient sources of magnesium, a mineral important to the conversion of sugar into energy. Citrus fruits contain natural sugars that provide a much steadier and more effective boost than the sugars used in processed foods. Keeping a bowl of nuts on the table and some citrus in the fridge is an excellent idea for the worker looking to gain some motivation in the morning.

3) Cut down on the coffee.

Coffee is an essential for most people to be able to remotely function in the morning. Some of us drink five or six cups throughout the course of a single day. The dominance of Starbucks and other coffee shop chains is a testament to our love for this beverage.

However, too much of a good thing is a bad thing, and this proverb holds especially true in the case of coffee. While coffee is healthy in small doses and does provide an excellent and quick boost, drinking too much coffee in the morning can lead to a serious crash by noon. Caffeine is a drug, and it must be treated as such. One cup of coffee in the morning, paired with a light and balanced breakfast, should be sufficient to give you the energy you'll need to attack the rest of the day.

The next time you wake up, don't ignore the first meal of the day. Give yourself some time to make a light, balanced, and nutritious breakfast. You won't regret it.

TIP #20: HOW TO BECOME
A RAW VEGAN IN 5 STEPS

Many people have done research regarding the raw vegan lifestyle and are interested in changing their diets. The problem that creeps up, however, is that going from a standard Western diet to a raw vegan diet can seem like a daunting task, and if you try to do it all at once, it is. That's why it's important to gradually ease into your new lifestyle and take it bit by bit. Below is a five-step guide outlining, in order, the things you should eliminate from your diet, one at a time. If you've gone without sugar for a week and you feel ready to take the next step, great; if you want to wait a month, great. This is your journey and it's up to you, but by following this order you can become a raw vegan with as minimal stress to your body as possible. If you only want to go vegan, you can stop at step four.

Step 1: Eliminate Sugar
Refined sugar is the single worst ingredient you're consuming. Not only does refined and processed sugar have literally no place in a healthy diet, your body doesn't know how to process it, so it can cause many side effects. The first step on your journey to raw veganism is to eliminate all refined sugar.

Step 2: Eliminate Processed Foods
For the purposes of your transition, processed foods essentially means anything in a package. This category includes chips, canned goods, packaged goods, and the like. However, at this point, it does not include meat, cheese, dried fruit, and things of that nature. You can still have those. A good tip is to stick to the outside of the grocery store. That's where the fruit, vegetables,

meat, bakery-fresh bread, and dairy are stored. All the processed foods are in the middle.

Step 3: Eliminate Meat

Meat is not only toxic to your body, but it's toxic to the environment, too. It has been estimated that 20 percent of the world's pollution is caused by the meat industry. Not only that, but most of commercialized meat includes additives, hormones, antibiotics, preservatives, and even gluten and wheat powder. Taking this step will not only save you a lot of calories and fat, but will be a major turning point on your road to becoming a raw vegan.

Step 4: Eliminate Dairy

Dairy is the logical elimination to make after you've become comfortable with your vegetarian lifestyle. When you eliminate dairy, know that this means the elimination of eggs, as well. At this point your diet will be made up of mostly fruits, vegetables, nuts, seeds, whole wheat pasta, vegan sauces, and the like. Once you've eliminated dairy, assuming you've followed the steps above, you are now a vegan. If you don't have any interest in becoming a raw vegan, that's completely fine; feel free to stop the transition right here. If you want to become a raw vegan, though, there is one more step you have to take.

Step 5: Eliminate Cooked Foods

When you cook your vegetables and food, you take what was a vibrant and living food and essentially kill it. You will notice that if you cook a bell pepper, that bright, green, beautiful food becomes the color of kelp or something similar. Cooking your food leeches the ingredients out of it, and many cooked foods, such as bread and pasta, are essentially paste made from wheat and water. Ever wonder where the words "pasta" and "pastry" come from? You will also need to eliminate oils, although some raw vegans do not; a low fat raw vegan, however, does eliminate oils. The choice is ultimately yours.

Final Destination

Congratulations! Once you've completed these steps, you have become a raw vegan. Hopefully this guide has served you well in helping you through the major milestones on your way to a healthier and more abundant life. The raw vegan lifestyle is beautiful, abundant, energizing, and healthy. It's kind to your body, your mind, your spirit, and the environment, as well as other living creatures. If it takes you a month or five years to get through the steps, it doesn't matter; the important thing is that you have taken steps consistently towards a healthier and cleaner way of living.

TIP #21: BECOMING A VEGETARIAN: WHAT YOU NEED TO KNOW

Are you thinking about changing your diet to eat less meat, or to exclude it altogether? If so, you're following in the footsteps of thousands of people who have enjoyed healthier lives. But becoming a vegetarian means more than turning your back on bacon sandwiches; you need to know what you should be eating, not just what you should be giving up.

If you're a meat eater now, think about your diet; it may be pretty healthy already, or there might be some room for improvement. Everything you eat and drink has an effect on your body. If you're going to exclude some of the things that are good for you, you'll need to replace them. That means identifying what you gain from meat products, and then finding a vegetarian alternative.

For most people, the meat in a meal is primarily there as a source of protein, and the vegetables are there to provide carbohydrates, fiber, and some minerals. If you take away the meat, you'll need to find an alternative source of protein. Unless you're taking the extra step to become a vegan, you'll still be able to eat eggs and dairy products, which are rich in protein. You can also get protein from nuts and seeds, soy and soy products, and beans and lentils. Although the vegetarian alternatives contain less protein, weight for weight, than meat, you won't need to be eating huge piles of lentils; 6 ounces of plain Greek yogurt and 4 ounces of tofu contain more protein together than 4 ounces of chicken breast.

In general, you'll need 1/2 to 1 gram of protein per pound of body weight, depending on your activity level. So if you weigh 140 pounds, you'll need between 70 and 140 grams of protein a day. The simplest way to make sure you're getting this from a vegetarian diet is to have a good source of protein at every meal. Remember: unless you are currently having meat at every meal, becoming vegetarian isn't just about replacing the meat with extra vegetables; you've got to be thinking "protein" at every mealtime.

Meat and fish are also good sources of minerals such as iron, zinc, iodine, and calcium. Your body needs iron for hemoglobin, so that your bloodstream can carry oxygen to your cells. If you're low on iron (anemic), you'll feel constantly lethargic and lacking in energy. If you don't get enough zinc, your immune system doesn't work properly, and you'll get ill more easily and take longer to get well. Iodine helps to regulate your metabolism, and calcium is essential for strong bones and healthy teeth. You can take supplements if you're concerned that you're not getting enough of these minerals, but you can get all you need from food.

Whole grains, nuts, and wheat germ will provide you with zinc, which is also found in cheese. If you like sushi, the seaweed wrapped around it is a source of iodine, but the easiest way to get iodine is to use iodized salt, which provides a good dose in less than a 1/2 teaspoon. Dark green vegetables like broccoli and kale are high in calcium, and of course milk and dairy products are full of it. Your body can't absorb calcium without vitamin D, so look for dairy products that are fortified with vitamin D, and look for fortified juices, soy products, and eggs. Those same dark green vegetables contain iron, which you can also find in whole grains and dried fruit and pulses. Your body needs vitamin C to absorb iron, so make sure you're combining these foods with plenty of citrus fruit, blueberries, sweet potatoes, and tomatoes.

The vitamin that you're most likely to miss out on when you give up meat is vitamin B12. This is needed for proper formation of red blood cells and to keep your nervous system functioning properly. A lack of vitamin B12 can lead to an inability to think clearly, and changes in personality such as irritability or depression. B12 is only found in meat and meat products, so as a vegetarian you'll need to get it from milk and dairy produce or from vegetarian foods that are specifically fortified with vitamin B12. Again, you might want to consider taking a supplement if you're not sure you can get enough from your diet. The good news is that there are no harmful effects in otherwise healthy people if you take more vitamin B12 than you need.

Nutritionists recommend eating two portions of oily fish per week, mainly because it's a great source of essential fatty acids (Omega-3), which are proven to help prevent heart disease and control inflammation. If you're giving up fish as well as meat, you'll need to find another source. Walnuts are high in Omega-3, and some eggs are specifically fortified with it. You can also find it in flax seeds, soy beans, and some soy products such as tofu.

It's easy to define a vegetarian as a person who doesn't eat meat. If you're making the shift to vegetarianism, you need to move beyond this definition. Stop focusing on what you don't eat, and start considering what you do eat. Becoming a vegetarian, whether for ethical, environmental, or health reasons, doesn't mean you'll miss out on any of the nutrients your body needs. But becoming a vegetarian does mean you'll need to change your thinking, not just your diet.

TIP #22: FIVE INGREDIENTS IN YOUR BREAKFAST THAT SHOULD BE AVOIDED AT ALL COSTS

A harmful consequence is the last thing someone expects when eating, especially when it's from the most important meal of the day. However, there are many people out there experiencing unhealthy and even life threatening problems because of the food they're consuming. Knowledge is indeed power, and hopefully with knowledge, health problems that can be easily avoided will decline.

What ingredients should be avoided then?
1. Used in jet fuel and embalming fluid, an ingredient commonly referred to as BHT, Butylated Hydroxytoluene is found in many processed foods and is a widely used preservative in many breakfast foods. BHT is used to stop oxidation in foods; however, it has been found to cause liver damage and increase the risk of cancer.

2. When one thinks of beetles, it's usually not in regards to food. Yet beetles are exactly what many people are eating on a daily basis. Made from dried red beetles, carmine is a red paste commonly found in some yogurts, as well as candy and fruit drinks. Carmine was found to cause anaphylaxis and other severe allergic reactions in some people.

3. A carcinogenic found in packaged meat, such as bacon and ham, sodium nitrite creates compounds that have the ability to cause cancer. These dangerous compounds, known as

nitrosamines, come about when sodium nitrite meets extremely high temperatures and highly acidic conditions such as the stomach.

4. Yellow #5, otherwise known as tartrazine, is commonly found in jam and many types of cereal. Many allergic reactions have been caused by this food coloring and it's believed to cause hyperactive behavior in children as well. Some studies have also linked yellow #5 to anxiety, migraines, clinical depression, and more.

5. Many people have heard of MSG and know to stay away from foods that have it. However, it's not widely known that MSG is labeled under different names to hide the fact that it's used in certain foods. Modified cornstarch, textured soy protein concentrate, and maltodextrin are just some of the names MSG has, which has been linked to a variety of ailments, such as migraines, seizures, skin rashes, and many more.

TIP #23: TWELVE HIGH PROTEIN SNACKS TO SATISFY YOUR HUNGER

Many dieters avoid red meat and other protein-rich foods when they are trying to lose weight, but that is not always a smart move. While cutting the amount of fat you consume makes sense, you still need plenty of protein to give you energy and keep you moving.

Exercise is just as important to your weight loss goal. Eating foods that are rich in protein and low in fat is one of the best ways to boost your energy and make you feel great. Just pack a few of these great high protein foods to enjoy throughout the day.

- **Almonds** - nuts are rich sources of protein, but almonds are particularly good when you are dieting. Almonds are filling, high in protein and rich in healthy Omega-3 fatty acids. Putting the cookie jar away and replacing it with a bowl of healthy almonds is a great way to avoid temptation and lose more weight.

- **Cottage cheese** - cottage cheese is one of the healthiest dairy product you can eat when you are on a diet. Mix your favorite fruits with a bowl of cottage cheese and enjoy a healthy snack at home or at work.

- **Pumpkin seeds** - pumpkin seeds are very rich in protein, making them a great pick me up at the office or at home. You can roast your own pumpkin seeds at home or buy ready-made versions at your favorite grocery store or organic market.

- Trail mix - trail mix is not just for hikers anymore. These delicious mixtures of nuts, dried fruit and seeds are perfect snacks for any time of day. Trail mix is particularly good as a post-workout snack. It is easy to transport and easy to snack on as you chat with your friends at the gym.

- Organic peanut butter - you probably already know that peanut butter is rich in protein, but you may not realize how versatile this simple food can be. You can enjoy peanut butter on whole wheat crackers, slathered on celery or even mixed into your favorite post-workout shake or smoothie.

- Hard boiled eggs - you do not have to avoid eggs when you are dieting. In fact, eggs should be a regular part of your diet. Hard boiled eggs are particularly well suited for snacking. They are easy to prepare and easy to take with you wherever you go.

- Oatmeal - a bowl of oatmeal is a great snack at the office and very easy to prepare. You can also enjoy a low-fat oatmeal muffin or even an oatmeal raisin cookie or two for a sweet treat.

- Hummus - hummus is a rich source of protein and delicious to boot. Enjoy hummus on a pita, or with your favorite flatbread or whole wheat bread. Keep a jar of hummus at your office and enjoy a delicious healthy snack any time the mood strikes.

- Tofu - enjoying a meatless meal once or twice a week is a great way to lose weight and lower your fat intake. Tofu is a great meat substitute for all your favorite dishes, so feel free to experiment and enjoy great vegetarian meals any time.

- Chocolate milk - quality dairy products should be part of your regular diet, and chocolate milk makes a great snack at home or at work. You can buy your favorite brand of chocolate milk at the store or choose a healthy dark chocolate cocoa powder and make your own.

- Homemade yogurt and berry parfait - yogurt makes a wonderful snack, and many office workers already enjoy it. Give your favorite office snack a new twist with a homemade yogurt and berry parfait. Just pick up some plain or vanilla yogurt, layer in your favorite fresh berries and enjoy.

- Black bean mini tacos - black beans are inexpensive to buy, easy to prepare and rich in protein. Perk up your workday with black bean mini tacos. Mini tacos are great snacks, and you can make enough to share with your coworkers.

TIP #24: SEVEN NUTRIENTS THAT YOUR DIET MAY BE MISSING

The human body is a compelling and amazing thing. Even the greatest scientists in the world have been completely baffled by the most basic functions of our bodies. For our bodies to be able to do the miraculous things that it does, we need to first give it the proper nutrients that it requires. Below are the seven nutrients that you probably are not getting enough of from your current diet.

1. Iron

The human body uses iron to carry oxygen from the lungs to the rest of the body. Iron is also used to help the muscles store and use oxygen. The human body needs just the right amount of iron, and it can be detrimental if your body has too much or too little.

How to get more Iron: Go see your doctor before you try to incorporate an iron supplement into your diet. Your physician will be able to tell you whether or not you need more iron. If you are looking to increase your consumption of iron there are a number of foods that are rich in this great nutrient. Try eating egg yolks, liver, dried fruits, and artichokes.

2. Vitamin D

Vitamin D is a special nutrient because it is the only vitamin that our bodies can consume and make. Our bodies make vitamin D by processing sunlight. Vitamin D regulates cell growth, maintains the optimal level of calcium, and is used to reduce inflammation and pain. If you have a Vitamin D deficiency, you may suffer from severe asthma, cognitive impairment, rickets, cardiovascular disease, and an increased risk of cancer.

How to get more Vitamin D: Eating a diet rich in vitamin D and getting enough exposure to the sun are the best ways to obtain more vitamin D. Foods that are rich in vitamin D include canned salmon, oysters, caviar, eggs, ham, salami, mushrooms, and sausages.

3. Calcium

Calcium is an essential nutrient that our bodies need to function properly. In fact, there is more calcium in your body than any other mineral. Calcium's main job is to make sure that your bones and teeth are healthy and strong. Other than strengthening bones, calcium is used to expand and contract blood vessels, send messages throughout the nervous system, and secrete hormones.

How to get more Calcium: Getting more calcium in your diet is easy. Simply change your diet to be higher in calcium. Some foods that are high in calcium include milk, cheese, yogurt, green vegetables, sardines, salmon, and spinach.

4. Fiber

The body uses fiber for proper digestion, the prevention of constipation, and the reduction of cholesterol levels. Fiber comes in two different types: soluble fiber and insoluble fiber. Soluble fiber reduces the amount of cholesterol and glucose in the blood. Insoluble fiber assists the body in proper digestion. Your body requires both types of fiber to run optimally. If your body is not getting enough fiber you will suffer from high blood pressure, diabetes, constipation, obesity, and cancer.

How to get more Fiber: The only way to get more fiber is to eat foods that are rich in fiber. Here are some foods that have high fiber content: prunes, pears, mangoes, raisins, rye, pecans, walnuts, navy beans, pinto beans, and kidney beans.

5. Vitamin B-12

Vitamin B-12 is a water soluble vitamin that is essential for the body to function properly. Vitamin B-12 cannot be made by humans, animals, or plants, but some types of bacteria are able to produce this amazing vitamin. Our bodies use vitamin B-12 for a variety of functions. The most important functions include, maintaining a healthy digestive system, converting carbohydrates into glucose, and maintaining the healthy regulation of our nervous systems. In addition, vitamin B-12 decreases the risk of breast cancer, colon cancer, lung cancer, and prostate cancer.

How to get more Vitamin B-12: The human body typically stores an adequate amount of vitamin B-12 in the liver, but with the typical modern diet most people are not getting enough of this vitamin. Try eating foods that are rich in vitamin B-12, such as, shellfish, eggs, and different types of cheeses.

6. Magnesium

Magnesium is an essential nutrient that is required for the human body to function properly. For instance, magnesium is used in over 300 chemical reactions throughout the body. Magnesium assists a number of systems and organs in the body, such as, the cardiovascular system, the nervous system, the digestive system, muscular system, excretory system, the immune system, and hormone-secreting glands. There are many uncomfortable side effects that coincide with a magnesium deficiency. For example, if you have a magnesium deficiency, you may experience headaches, weight gain, depression, nausea, seizure, vomiting, and an increased heart rate.

How to get more Magnesium: There are many foods that are rich in magnesium. Some examples of foods that are rich in magnesium include spinach, pumpkin seeds, brown rice, soybeans, halibut, dried figs, and bananas.

7. Potassium

Potassium enables muscles and nerves to communicate. Additionally, it regulates our body's water balance by moving nutrients in cells and waste out of cells. If you develop a potassium deficiency, you will experience terrible side effects, such as, muscle cramps, fatigue, and constipation.

How to get more Potassium: Getting more potassium in your diet can be easy, and it just requires you to eat a diet higher in Potassium. There are a number of foods that are rich in potassium, such as spinach, collards, carrots, potatoes, grapes, bananas, grapefruits, and oranges.

TIP #25: THE BENEFITS
OF HERBAL TEA

Herbal tea has become extremely popular with Westerners taking a more holistic approach to health care. With herbal tea, you are actually drinking herbal infusions, also known as a tisane, rather than actual brewed teas. Like normal tea, herbal teas are made with near-boiling water but they do not come from the Camellia sinensis bush that all tea comes from.

Herbal teas have been used for centuries, especially in the East, for the multitude of medicinal qualities that they possess. There are a plethora of teas available in vibrant colors, flavorful tastes and pleasant fragrances. Some of the general benefits of herbal tea include: reducing anxiety, supporting heart health, alleviating stomach problems, providing cleansing properties for the body and promoting energy and vitality.

Herbal infusions can contain a variety of ingredients from dried leaves, dried fruit, flowers, grasses, seeds and bark. Commercial fruit teas such as Rosehip are generally blended for flavor from artificial ingredients. They offer little to no health benefits whereas herbal teas usually contain real herbs and should be the tea of choice for the health-savvy tea-drinker. For an effective remedy, drink your preferred cup of herbal tea 3-4 times a day. When it comes to store-bought tea, try to buy organic. But teas made from organic leaves are more effective than ground tea bags. It's important to remember not to let water reach boiling point when heating it, as the heat will kill the nutrients in the leaves.

The following is a list of herbal teas and their medicinal effects:
- **Chamomile** fights mild anxiety, is an anti-inflammatory, an anti-spasmodic and great for treating mild insomnia.

- **Fennel** is a wonderful digestive aid and also a diuretic that helps clean the kidneys and rid the body of toxins.

- **Ginger** is used to treat nausea; colds, indigestion, headaches, circulation and can help fight infection in its early stages.

- **Ginseng** gives energy and vitality to the body and serves to lift moods.

- **Hibiscus** reduces high blood pressure and relieves menstrual cramps.

- **Green Tea** speeds up metabolism thereby aiding weight loss. It's also high in antioxidants and helps in tissue regeneration. This, in turn protects against aging.

- Slippery Elm is a bark that relieves stomach cramps and other gastro-intestinal issues such as indigestion.

- **Peppermint** is an effective "stomach healer" as it alleviates stomach cramps, Irritable Bowel Syndrome and gallstone problems. Peppermint also strengthens the immune system and boosts mental power.

TIP #26: SEVEN HEALTHY, ALL-NATURAL ALTERNATIVES TO SUGAR

For anyone seeking to slim down or get more fit, cutting out processed sugars is no-brainer. However, ditching sugar and high fructose corn syrup doesn't mean that you can't enjoy a sweet treat: there are several natural alternative sweeteners that can provide the same flavors without all of the calories and empty carbs. Below are the best of the best when it comes to alternative sweetener options.

Stevia:

Used as a sweetener for centuries in South America, stevia is an herb that is much sweeter than sugar. Stevia is an enormously popular sugar alternative due to the fact that it has zero calories and no glycemic impact, making it the perfect choice for diabetics as well as anyone that wants to lose inches from their waist.

Xylitol:

A common ingredient in sugar-free chewing gum, xylitol is a low-calorie sweetener that can help fight the growth of bacteria. Xylitol is much sweeter than sugar, meaning that you don't need to use nearly as much of it. Xylitol is best used for adding to coffee or tea rather than large-scale applications like baking, as ingesting too much xylitol can cause an upset stomach.

Honey:

While it isn't calorie-free, honey is still a healthier option than processed sugars. Honey has a significantly lower glycemic index, meaning it causes less of a blood sugar spike and is less likely to result in a "crash" after consumption. As an added bonus, honey is packed with potent antioxidants, and locally-sourced honey can even help treat allergies.

Monk Fruit Extract:

A granulated sweetener derived from a species of sweet melon, monk fruit extract is still relatively uncommon despite being used as an herbal remedy throughout Southeast Asia for centuries. One of the primary benefits of monk fruit extract is that it lacks the bitter aftertaste that some people experience with other sugar alternatives.

Coconut Sugar:

Coconut sugar is has seen a recent boost in popularity, and for good reason. Made by evaporating coconut sap, this sweetener has a rich taste similar to brown sugar. Coconut sugar also boasts a low glycemic index, and it can be substituted in a 1:1 ratio for processed sugars in virtually any recipe.

Agave Nectar:

Agave nectar contains more calories than sugar by weight, but it can be used in smaller amounts because it is much sweeter. Agave nectar is digested and converted to glucose more slowly than sugar and high fructose corn syrup, which means that it has a more mild effect on blood sugar and results in less of a sugary "buzz." Agave nectar is perfect for use in coffee or tea, but should be avoided for baking purposes.

Maple Syrup:

Like agave nectar and honey, maple syrup takes the body longer to break down, resulting in a lower glycemic impact and less of a strain on your energy levels. For maximum benefit, look for darker syrup, which contains more antioxidants and nutrients than lighter shades of syrup.

Healthy eating doesn't mean that you have to give up on sweets. Swapping out processed sugar and high fructose corn syrup for some of the all-natural alternative options on this list can help anyone trim down and achieve their own personal fitness or weight loss goals.

TIP #27: EAT THESE 10 FOODS TO BOOST YOUR IMMUNE SYSTEM

Can what you eat help build up your resistance to disease and infections? Several recent studies suggest that the antioxidants, vitamins and minerals in some foods can help your immune system perform at peak efficiency.

What does this mean? Fewer colds for one thing. As kids go back to school and we spend more time indoors in recirculated air, exposure to germs rises. And if you do get a cold or even the flu, a high-functioning immune system means shorter duration and less severity of your illness.

With that in mind, look for opportunities to include these foods in your diet:

1. Broccoli
Broccoli is an easy superfood to embrace. Abundant year round and inexpensive, broccoli contains vitamin A and vitamin C, and at least one study has shown broccoli to stimulate the immune systems of mice. Broccoli is delicious in stir fries or as a simple side dish with some cheese grated on top.

2. Sweet Potatoes
Sweet potatoes are another low-cost immune booster. Rich in the antioxidant beta carotene, sweet potatoes also have a lot of vitamin A, which may lower the risk of some cancers. Sweet potatoes can substitute for regular potatoes as a mealtime staple-- serve them baked, mashed, or look for sweet potato fries in the

grocery freezer.

3. Tea

Black or green, caffeinated or decaf, tea provides a potent dose of polyphenols and flavonoids. These antioxidants destroy free radicals, which damage and age your body. Drink iced tea in warm weather, and hot tea in cool seasons.

4. Mushrooms

The humble mushroom is more potent than you might think. Mushrooms have selenium, a trace element that has been linked to less severity in flu infections. Mushrooms are also a good source of B vitamins, important to a healthy immune system, and some animal studies have shown mushrooms to have anti-viral effects. You don't need fancy gourmet mushrooms, either--the common button mushroom is just as nourishing. Mush-rooms can go into all kinds of dishes--salads, soups, sauces and gravies, stir fries, and even as a sandwich topping.

5. Watermelon

Watermelon is a great source of glutathione, an antioxidant known to be an immune system booster. The red pulp closest to the rind has the most glutathione, so when eating watermelon be sure to eat all the way to the edge! Watermelon is a refreshing addition to a fruit salad, and is delicious eaten on its own.

6. Cabbage

Cabbage is inexpensive and easy to find throughout the winter months when other veggies become scarcer and pricier. Cabbage contains the antioxidant glutamine as well as anthocyanins, which protect the brain from the plaques that cause Alzheimers, and lower the risk of diabetes. In winter months, cabbage is a delicious addition to soups and stews, while in the summertime, coleslaw made from cabbage and chilled is a cool treat.

7. Almonds

Almonds are a nutrition powerhouse--just one quarter of a cup contains more than half the daily recommended allowance of vitamin E, an immune system booster. Almonds also contain a number of B vitamins, which seem to have some effect on helping your systems bounce back from the effects of stress. A handful of almonds makes an energizing and filling afternoon snack, or try almond milk in the place of regular milk on your breakfast cereal.

8. Yogurt

Choose low fat yogurt that contains live cultures to add some probiotics to your diet. Some research evidence suggests that probiotics give a powerful push to the immune system. Yogurt also has vitamin D. Low levels of vitamin D have been linked to a higher severity in colds and flu. Yogurt is another healthy snack to reach for, or mix granola and fruit into some yogurt for a healthy breakfast.

9. Spinach

Spinach is high in folate, which helps your body repair DNA and produce new cells. A potent mix of fiber, antioxidants, and vitamins, spinach has rightly been called a "superfood." Spinach is most nutritious eaten raw or very lightly cooked. Eat raw spinach in salads or on top of sandwiches; stir some spinach into a stir fry or pasta dish as the very end of cooking, and allow the heat of the food to wilt it.

10. Garlic

Garlic was known to the Chinese, Egyptian, Greek and Roman civilizations as a medicinal herb. Garlic acts as an antibiotic, killing bacteria that cause infections, especially the bacteria H. pylori, which is linked to both ulcers and some types of stomach cancer. Garlic is a tasty addition to many dishes. To get the most effect, peel and chop garlic and then let it sit for 15-20 minutes before adding it in cooking. This allows the enzymes in garlic to fully activate, making it as potent as possible.

TIP #28: HEALTH BENEFITS YOU GET WHEN YOU EAT FIBER

You have probably heard that fiber is good for your health. Well it is and you are about to learn why. Fiber is a combination of different substances found in plants. It comes in the form of soluble fiber and insoluble fiber, both of which keep your health in good shape. The difference between the two is soluble fiber melts into a fluid when it is mixed with water, but insoluble fiber is not affected by water this way. When soluble fiber is consumed, it transforms into a tacky substance that adheres to poisons and removes them from the body. Insoluble fiber goes right through the body when it is eaten, which is why it prevents constipation. Fiber has a number of other health benefits too.

Low Cholesterol

People who have an elevated LDL level may be able to bring their bad cholesterol down with the help of soluble fiber. With regular consumption, cholesterol can be reduced by 5 percent and up to 10 percent. Foods that contain a high amount of soluble fiber include oat bran, beans, lentils, oranges, grapefruit, peas, apples, and high-fiber cereal.

Regulation of Blood Sugar

People with diabetes have a high amount of sugar in their blood. Fortunately, increased fiber consumption can lower the amount of glucose going into the bloodstream. In order to get this health benefit from fiber, you should consume complex carbohydrate foods such as potatoes, whole grain pasta, brown rice, beans, barley, and oat bran. .

Protection From Cancer

Estrogen has been known to cause breast cancer, but a diet that is made up of plenty of fiber-filled fruits and vegetables like apples, bananas, broccoli, Brussels sprouts, cabbage, cauliflower, and carrots lowers a woman's level of blood estrogen. Whole wheat breads and cereals as well as whole grains also bring the level down. Fiber offers protection from endometrial and colon cancer too, and men who eat plenty of fiber have a reduced risk of developing prostate cancer.

Relief From Intestinal Disorders

People who have diverticular disease can turn to fiber for relief. When there is a lot of fiber in the diet, the fiber absorbs water and acts as a stool softener. This makes bowel movements regular and abdominal cramps less painful. Those who suffer from irritable bowel syndrome or a mild case of inflammatory bowel disease can also get relief from constipation and diarrhea with the help of fiber. Your doctor will be able to tell you just how much fiber you need.

Weight Loss

Since there's such a small amount of calories in fiber, and because fiber gives you a feeling of fullness, losing weight is an easy thing to do when you put fiber in your diet. Another great weight-loss feature fiber has is it cannot be digested. Eat more fiber foods if you want to lose weight and for all the other reasons mentioned.

The amount of fiber that is recommended to be eaten every day is 25 grams minimum, but don't start eating that amount right away because you could get cramps, flatulence, bloating, and diarrhea if you do. Add fiber to your diet slowly, and if you feel any adverse reactions, consult with your doctor. What's also important when you consume fiber is to drink between 64 to 80 ounces of water a day. Without enough water to hydrate the fiber in your body, you could become constipated.

TIP #29: SEVEN TIPS FOR APPETITE CONTROL

Food cravings come without warning and are often difficult to resist. Your appetite may seem out of control, but you are stronger than a feeling. Following a few tips will help you tame your hunger.

1.   Eat breakfast every day. Skipping meals will not help you lose or maintain weight. Three well-balanced meals and one healthy afternoon snack is recommended to keep your appetite at bay. Space meals from four to five hours apart to keep blood sugar levels stable.

2.   Healthy snacks can include raw veggies and hummus dip, a small handful of nuts, hard-boiled egg, and pumpkin seeds. Eat slowly to allow time for your brain to get the message that you are full. Avoid sweetened snacks, such as honey-roasted almonds or chocolate-covered raisins.

3.   Keep a water container at your desk when you are at work. Staying hydrated keeps your appetite satisfied between meals. Drink only water or sparkling water, and avoid energy drinks and juices.

4.   Have an appetizer of fiber-rich vegetables before starting your meal. Because the fiber is filling, you will not eat as much. Try to include some raw vegetables for lunch and dinner. Satisfying your appetite at mealtime reduces the desire for snacking.

5.   If you're feeling hungry between meals, enjoy a cup of hot

tea. Herbal or regular are both acceptable, but avoid adding sugar of any kind.

6.   Regular exercise reduces the risk of overeating. Exercise increases the level of appetite-suppressing peptide YY.

7.   Adding a little organic red cider vinegar to your food lowers the glycemic index and causes your food to metabolize more slowly. Cinnamon also slows the metabolic rate and can be added to coffee, tea, smoothies, stew, and chili.

Following these seven tips will help keep your appetite in check. Add them to your daily routine. Healthy foods keep you satisfied and help you reach and maintain your weight goal.

TIP #30: FOUR HEALTHY SNACKS TO KEEP AT THE OFFICE

Modern offices are a prime location for unhealthy, high-calorie snacks. Between the vending machine stocked with junk food and soda, the giant bowl of candy at reception, and the never-ending parade of birthday cakes in the break room, every work day in a typical office is chock full of temptation. When you forget your lunch or that afternoon slump hits, you may find yourself reaching for a sugar or junk food fix without even thinking about it.

Those empty calories can really add up, and can easily lead to weight gain. You don't have to succumb to temptation, though. Try keeping a few non-perishable, healthy snacks stashed in your office or desk drawer. The next time you find yourself working through lunch or struggling through a mid-afternoon crash, reach for these healthy options instead of noshing on junk.

- **Nuts** - Nuts provide a quick boost of energy via their fat content. They're also loaded with protein and fiber, which will helps you feel fuller longer. Nuts are a great source of several nutrients like vitamin E, potassium, and magnesium, too. Avoid salted or honey-roasted nuts when you can, opting for raw or toasted nuts instead.

- **Salmon or tuna pouches & whole wheat crackers** - Salmon & tuna are great sources of protein, while the whole wheat crackers are a great source of carbohydrate. This combination will fill you up and keep you feeling full more than a slice of birthday cake or potato chips from the vending machine ever could. The fish also provide an added bonus to your health in the form of Omega-3 fatty acids.

- **Fruit** - While not all fruits can be kept at room temperature for very long, fruits like apples, pears, oranges, and bananas should stay fresh for at least the length of an average work week. Low-sugar fruit cups or applesauce are great non-perishable alternatives to fresh fruit. Apples and pears are particularly excellent sources of fiber, so they're generally the most filling options, but any fruit that you like to eat will make a fine choice.

- **Protein bars** - While some protein bars are actually higher in calories and sugar than an average candy bar, they are incredibly convenient as they will stay fresh in their packaging for months. They can still work as a healthy snack if you choose wisely: Avoid protein bars high in sugar and calories. Also, you'd be surprised how many products marketed as "protein bars" are actually very low in protein, so make sure you select a high-protein variety to help yourself feel full.

Everyone gets hungry at work from time to time, but it can sometimes seem impossible to find healthy choices to satisfy your hunger. You shouldn't ever have to worry about finding a healthy snack option at work. Try keeping nuts, salmon or tuna pouches with whole wheat crackers, fruit, and protein bars on hand, and you'll always have a healthy snack option at the ready.

TIP #31: BENEFITS OF LEMONS AND LIMES

Lemons and limes are citrus fruits that are filled with vitamins, minerals and health benefits. These fruits are excellent sources of Vitamin C, Vitamin B6, potassium, calcium, magnesium, folic acid and flavonoids. These vitamins and minerals are necessary for optimum health. For instance, potassium is important for the brain and nervous system to function properly. Magnesium is needed for the heart to remain healthy. Vitamin C helps promote a strong immune system.

Lemons and limes have antiviral and antibacterial properties. They also contain phytochemicals that have antibiotic and anti-cancer effects. Lemons and limes have anti-inflammatory properties that can help reduce the inflammation of conditions such as arthritis and gout. These fruits can detoxify the body and purify the liver. Lemons and limes can also break down kidney stones and help prevent them.

These citrus fruits are good for digestion and healthy bowels too. Lemons and limes can aid the process of elimination and make bowel movements easier. Drinking a glass of warm lemon or lime water first thing in the morning helps relieve constipation. The fruits can also relieve indigestion, bloating and heartburn. Lime helps alleviate nausea and diarrhea as well.

The two fruits are very helpful for boosting immunity, and helping to prevent colds or flu. Lemons and limes help treat and prevent cough, sore throat and even ear infections. Including these fruits in your regular diet can easily help boost the power of your immune system. You can add lemons and limes to salads and desserts, use them in smoothies, or add them to a daily cup of tea. Lemons and limes have other benefits, such as lowering blood pressure, strengthening eyesight and treating dandruff. Although further research needs done, there is some speculation that the citrus fruits may even alleviate asthma.

Although lemons and limes share many of the same benefits, each fruit is individually beneficial. Lemons strengthen the blood vessels and reduce fluid retention by increasing urinary output. Limes are believed to aid respiratory disorders, and may be particularly useful to those who suffer from conditions such as asthma.

Although lemon is considered safe for pregnant and breastfeeding women when used as a normal part of the diet, lime should be avoided since there is not enough known about its effects. Lime may interact with medications that need to be broken down by the liver, or that increase sensitivity to sunlight. It is best to consult with a physician before taking supplements or making any changes to your regular diet, especially if you have an existing health condition.

TIP #32: FIVE LEAFY GREEN VEGETABLES YOU NEED IN A HEALTHY DIET

As children, we were often told to eat our vegetables. As adults, it's even more important to eat our daily intake of vegetables (6-9 servings per day), especially green vegetables. Leafy green vegetables are packed with healthy vitamins, minerals, and anti-oxidants that can ward off disease and illness. According to a study in the British Medical Journal, leafy green vegetables may lower the risk of type 2 diabetes by 14 percent.

When picking out leafy vegetables in the store or at a farmer's market, stick with dark green leaves - darker leaves contain more nutrients. The following five leafy green vegetables pack a punch, and add much-needed fiber and nutritional benefits to your diet. If you aren't a fan of eating leafy greens by themselves, add them to smoothies blended with fruit, for sweetness. Raw green smoothies help detoxify the body, and give you an energy boost throughout your day.

Microgreens

Microgreens are the underdeveloped shoots of vegetables (such as cabbage, arugula, and cilantro). A 2012 study by the U.S. Department of Agriculture reports that microgreens have nutrient levels up to six times greater than mature plants. Microgreens contain vitamin K, vitamin E, beta-carotene, and lutein. By adding microgreens to your salad, you can reduce cancer risk and improve skin and eye health.

Kale

Kale is often called a superfood because of its powerful phyton-utrients. This curly leafy green vegetable contains lutein, an antioxidant that aids in better vision and protects the eyes. It also contains vitamin C, beta-carotene, and cancer-fighting sulforaphane and glucosinolate. Kale also has anti-inflammatory properties and antioxidants, including 45 different flavonoids.

Spinach
Dark leafy spinach is chock full of vitamins and minerals, including magnesium and potassium. It is also an excellent source of iron and protein. Look for darker spinach leaves because they have a higher concentration of vitamin C (compared to lighter leaves). By eating spinach, you can help reduce blood glucose levels, lower blood pressure, and improve bone health. Spinach also protects the digestive tract from inflammation.

Swiss Chard
Swiss chard tastes mildly bitter, but the nutritional benefits far outweigh its taste. It contains a range of vitamins and minerals including vitamins C and A, and potassium, iron, and magnesium. Swiss chard also provides 300% of the daily recommended value of vitamin K. In order to neutralize chard's bitter taste, sauté or lightly steam when preparing it.

Romaine Lettuce
Skip the iceberg lettuce when making salads and replace with Romaine lettuce instead. Iceberg contains mostly water and does not have any nutritional value, while Romaine is high in vitamins A and C. One head of Romaine contains more vitamin C than one orange (167% RDA). If you are watching your weight, one cup of Romaine lettuce is only 10 calories. It is also rich in B-vitamins such as folate, thiamine, riboflavin, niacin, pantothenic acid, and pyridoxine.

Whenever possible, buy organic green leafy vegetables, to avoid toxic pesticide residue on greens, or grow your own. By adding green leafy vegetables to your meals, your diet will be packed with rich vitamins and minerals to support overall good health.

TIP #33: FIVE REASONS
TO EAT BROWN RICE
INSTEAD OF WHITE

Anyone who knows how to cook white rice can prepare brown rice just as easily by allowing a little more time. Nature's colors rarely include white, but the milling process for rice removes its brown tone as well as its nutritional elements. Brown rice is not refined, allowing it to retain its essential nutrients.

Removing the nutrition contained in the nutrient-rich germ and bran requires rice manufacturers to fortify white rice with B vitamins and iron to restore some of its food value. Brown rice contains vitamin E, a nutrient not found in white rice. Using brown rice instead of white can reduce the risk of developing Type 2 diabetes, according to WebMD, and it can aid in the prevention of other diseases as well. In its natural state, rice is a whole grain like oatmeal, barley, whole wheat, bulgar, and popcorn.

Getting Better Nutrition

The benefits of brown rice are far superior to those found in the modified and fortified rice product that is the most familiar form of the grain, including these:

1. Fiber content

The outer hull of the brown rice grain is the only part that is removed in milling, leaving the fiber rich bran and germ. The Mayo Clinic's list of high fiber foods shows that one cup of brown rice contains 3.5 grams of fiber, and white rice has less than half as much. A diet that is high in fiber improves the function of the digestive tract, and it may reduce the incidence of health problems such as diabetes, heart disease and obesity. Women need at least 21 grams of fiber daily, and men need upwards of 30.

2. Blood sugar stabilization

Risk of diabetes diminishes with the regular consumption of a half cup of brown rice every day by helping to stabilize glucose levels in blood. Food that scores low on the glycemic index (GI) digests slowly and provides an even flow of glucose instead of a sharp increase. Food that is high on the index produces quick bursts of energy soon after they are consumed, resulting in a drop in blood glucose level that allows hunger to occur again. Brown rice has a GI rating that is more than 10 points lower than white rice, according to reports from the Harvard Medical School.

3. Resistance to illness

Selenium is a mineral that is found in soil and water, finding its way into whole food grains. Brown rice contains more than 27 percent of the daily requirement for adults while white rice provides only 17 percent. The mineral is associated with a reduced risk of developing arthritis, heart disease and cancer. Manganese in a cup of brown rice satisfies 80 percent of the daily requirement for adults, benefiting the reproductive and nervous system while also helping to synthesize fats. The body uses potassium to synthesize proteins and to maintain a proper fluid balance, and white as well as brown rice contains one percent or less of the daily requirement.

Brightly colored fruits and vegetables are usually recognized as sources of antioxidants, but brown rice contains them as well. Antioxidants are valuable for repairing cells that are damaged by air pollution and substandard diets as well as for reducing the risk of developing heart disease. Researchers at the Harvard School of Public Health reported a higher risk of Type 2 diabetes among a test group of health professionals who ate white rice and a reduced risk by those who ate brown rice at least twice a week.

4. Bone health

The National Institutes of Health (NIH) cites the importance of magnesium in the development of bones and in producing a normal heart rhythm, conduction of nerve impulses, and contraction of muscles. The Office of Dietary Supplements at NIH confirms that refining rice substantially lowers its magnesium content. The body depends on magnesium for nerve and muscle functions, control of glucose levels, and regulation of blood pressure. Up to 60 percent of magnesium in the body resides in bones, and most of the remainder is contained in soft tissue.

Low intake of magnesium increases the risk of developing some types of illness over time, including cardiovascular disease, hypertension, Type 2 diabetes, osteoporosis, and migraine headaches. A serving of brown rice contains 84 milligrams of magnesium while white rice contains only 6. The recommended allowance for women is 320 and 420 for men, with one cup providing 20 percent of daily magnesium requirements for men and 26 percent for women.

5. Taste, consistency, and eye appeal

The colorful appearance of brown rice complements a plate, and it pleases the palate. Its consistency is similar to al dente in pasta, providing some resistance that releases a deliciously nutty flavor. As a complex carbohydrate, it supplies energy in a tasty form. The grains tend to remain loose and separate more effectively than those in white rice, and it needs no butter or gravy to give it flavor.

Healthier and better tasting brown rice provides many health benefits that are not available in white rice. Unfamiliarity with cooking methods prevents some cooks from experimenting with it, but its appeal to young and old who are fitness and nutrition conscious is increasing its popularity.

TIP #34: FIVE DELICIOUS HEALTH BENEFITS OF GREEK YOGURT

Greek yogurt is known for its great taste and smooth texture, but it's also a wholesome health food. From a rich offering of nutrients to helping your digestive system, Greek yogurt can boost your health in multiple ways. Here's a look at five health benefits you can enjoy when you savor the delicious taste of Greek yogurt.

It's Full of Healthy Probiotics that Help Digestion

Your body, especially your digestive system, is naturally full of many different types of bacteria: some bad, others good. Many Greek yogurts contain these good bacteria, called probiotics, which help your health in a variety of ways. Probiotics aid digestive health by helping keep your digestion regular and preventing diarrhea. In addition, they can also alleviate the severity of some digestive conditions such as irritable bowel syndrome and Crohn's disease. Probiotics can also strengthen your immunity system. However, not all yogurts labeled as Greek actually contain probiotics. Look for yogurts that say contains live active cultures, not made with live active cultures, to ensure you're getting the benefits of probiotics.

It's High in Protein and Nutrients

Because of the way Greek yogurt is made, which involves straining the whey liquid from the yogurt, it contains much more protein than other types of yogurt. Greek yogurt typically contains between 13 and 20 grams of protein per cup, while conventional yogurt often only has 5 to 10 grams. Protein fights hunger and helps you feel satisfied for longer, and it's an essential nutrient for building muscle. Greek Yogurt is also high in a variety of other essential nutrients, including potassium, zinc, vitamin B6, and vitamin B12, as well as calcium, which improves bone strength.

It's Low in Sugar and Sodium

Most brands of plain Greek yogurt have around half the amount of sugar found in regular yogurt, which also means lower overall carbohydrates. Greek yogurts usually have around fifty milligrams of sodium, which is approximately half of what's found in regular yogurt. Because of its low sugar and carbs, Greek yogurt is a healthy choice for diabetics as a breakfast or snack food. But, beware that flavored or sweetened varieties contain way more sugar and carbohydrates.

It Can Help You Lose Weight

Greek yogurt is especially appealing to people looking to shed weight. Protein, which Greek yogurt is high in, takes longer to digest, helping you feel satisfied for longer. Since Greek yogurt is also low in carbs, it's a healthy, low-impact addition to a meal that helps you feel more satisfied, and a great snack to help take the edge off of your cravings. If you're conscious about weight-management, be sure to get plain, nonfat or low-fat varieties with no added sweetener or flavors.

It Can Help Lower Blood Pressure

Greek yogurt is high in calcium, magnesium and potassium, all important nutrients that have been linked to lower blood pressure and decreased risk of cardiac issues such as heart attack. The high amount of protein found in Greek yogurt also contributes to a healthy heart. Look for plain low-fat or nonfat variety for maximum health benefit.

With so many health benefits on tap, Greek yogurt's recent explosion in popularity has definitely happened for good reason.

However, not all Greek yogurts are created equal when it comes to healthiness. Flavored varieties and those with added sugar have higher sodium, sugar, and carbohydrates, which diminish health benefits. As mentioned before, look for " contains live active cultures" on the label to ensure you're getting the benefit of probiotics. Be a smart consumer and shop carefully, and then enjoy the tasty health benefits of Greek yogurt.

TIP #35: BENEFITS OF GOING ORGANIC: WHY YOU SHOULD EAT MORE ORGANIC FOOD

Organic food used to be considered a strange new concept, only eaten by people with picky or peculiar diets. Now organic food has hit the headlines, and more people are experimenting with the organic lifestyle. Are there any true differences between organic and non-organic produce besides the increased price tag? What are the benefits, if any?

Pesticides: What's the Truth?
Many farmers use pesticides to reduce the risk of contamination from pests, weeds and other potential carriers of disease. There are many types of pesticides, including: herbicides, insecticides, fungicides and disinfectants. These pesticides are easily absorbed into the food you will end up putting on your plate. Pesticides can potentially cause detrimental effects for humans, ranging from mild symptoms such as stomach pains and headaches, to serious health conditions such as cancer and infertility. Organic farmers do not use synthetic pesticides. Legally they must only use organic pesticides and natural methods for preventing contamination in order to classify their food as organic. Since organic food does not contain any unnatural substances, it is safer to consume than non-organic produce. Parents of babies and young children may opt for organically grown food as it reduces the chance of infection and illnesses, and also helps promote healthy development.

Genetically Modified Organisms (GMOs)
Why would farmers want to alter the natural growth of crops

and animals by genetically modifying them? Farmers want to increase productively, decrease growing time, and make their food appealing and attractive to consumers. Organic food is often more expensive because they allow nature to do the job alone, which takes time, patience, and sometimes undesirable results. It may not always look as colorful, perfectly shaped and appealing as non-organic alternatives, but wouldn't you want to pay just a little more money to eat food that's completely natural and won't be detrimental to your health?

Taste Testing: Does Organic Food Taste Better?
Non-organic food may win against organic food in a beauty contest, but it certainly won't win in a taste test. If you've ever tasted organic strawberries, for example, you'll know that they are often far superior in taste compared to genetically modified strawberries. Why do you think so many top chefs opt for organic food in their restaurants?

Sustainability
Organic farming aims to work with nature in order to grow food. It does not damage the earth and is an ecological way of growing and harvesting crops year after year. The chemicals used in non-organic farming can wear away soil, and remain in the earth for hundreds of years. More chemicals need to be created and distributed in order to replace the chemicals that become ineffective at preventing contamination, which is not sustainable farming. A healthy environment means healthy food and healthy people!

TIP #36: SOME KEY REASONS WHY PEOPLE FAST

Fasting is an approach to internal cleansing and healing that has its origins in antiquity. Ancient healers such as Hippocrates and Paracelsus believed that denying the body food for periods of time encouraged it to heal itself. Many fasts have been undergone for religious reasons as well – typically as a method of spiritual atonement or as a demonstration of devotion. Here we're going to explore the reasons why people fast for fitness and nutritional reasons.

In the modern day, fasts are often associated with bodily cleanses. Allowing your body to go without food for a few days actually flushes out your system because it has a chance to either burn or otherwise rid itself of unprocessed food. This oftentimes includes pollutants and other toxins. When your body doesn't have to work on digesting meals it can turn its energies towards other healing tasks.

Burning up lingering calories also accomplishes the elimination of toxins that may have been holing up within your system. This lends itself to internal balance and rejuvenation. During this process you may find your mental habits shifting towards more health-conscious motifs as well. Fasting makes your system particularly sensitive to anything that goes into it. You may discover an aversion to substances like caffeine and alcohol. Because fasting alters your cravings it can also make transitioning into a new diet much easier.

Much has been written about fasting. Some of this literature applauds the potential benefits while some of it warns of the possible dangers. Most people begin with a simple two-day fast to get themselves acclimated to the process. They may even allow themselves some nutrients by way of sipping juice or other liquids occasionally. This approach can achieve the same desired health benefits without putting as much stress on the body. Typically, though, your body will not be as taxed as you feel like it must be. It has storehouses of sugars and fats that it can draw upon for basic sustenance. Just be sure to stay well hydrated throughout the duration of any fast.

If you feel unsure about the safety of fasting but still long to try it, there are ways of doing it under supervision. Although conventional medicine does not support fasting as an approach to health, there are many homeopaths and naturopathic and ayurvedic doctors who make a practice of monitoring people who do this.

Sometimes people embark upon fasts for reasons that are neither medical nor strictly religious. They view it as a spiritual endeavor similar to Native American vision quests. The idea here is that turning one's attention away from the physical world (symbolized, in this case, by food) turns one's mind towards spiritual values and the larger entities of life. Our daily habits of filling ourselves at set mealtimes can lull our minds into a more mundane frame of reference. Fasting brings us into a more direct encounter with the bare facts of life. The experience can remind us of what is really important to us and what is merely peripheral.

TIP #37: FOOD AND DRINK - 5 EASY WAYS TO BOOST YOUR BRAIN POWER

Everything you eat has an effect on how you think, how you perform at work, how positive or negative you feel – on your entire life. Armed with the knowledge that your feelings and moods are in your own hands and not simply a reaction to external events, you can transform the way you think and act on a day-to-day basis. In today's fast-paced high tech world where everything has to be delivered instantly, it is difficult to keep up with the demands of a busy life. When tiredness takes over, brain power diminishes very quickly, so what can you do to give it a much-needed boost?

Increase your mental alertness with food and drink:

1. Protein
Protein maximises brain power and mental alertness, and by including some protein with every meal or snack you can reduce the soporific after-effects of eating carbohydrates.
In practical terms this could mean:
- Eating meat with your pasta
- Enjoying chicken on your bread roll
- Opting for good quality fish with your chips

Protein also keeps you feeling full for longer so there will be less likelihood of reaching for a chocolate bar when hit by the mid-afternoon slump. Good sources of protein include lean chicken, turkey and ham, fish, and eggs.

2. Dietary boron

Boron is a trace mineral that appears to have an effect on cognitive performance, including long-term and short-term memory, research suggests. A deficiency of boron can result in slower reaction times, memory impairment and a general lack of mental awareness.

Boron is present in many fruits, vegetables and nuts:
- Fruits, including apples, pears, peaches, and grapes
- Leafy vegetables
- Nuts, including almonds, Brazil nuts, hazelnuts and cashews

3. Oily fish
A great source of essential fatty acids (EFAs), oily fish such as salmon, kippers, pilchards and trout boost both memory and brain power. Results will not be noticed immediately, but if you regularly eat oily fish over a period of approximately 6 months, memory and mental alertness will improve.

Eating a 150g portion of salmon each week provides the recommended amount, so it will not be too hard on your wallet either.

White fish, although still a good source of protein, contains lower levels of DHA, an omega-3 fatty acid that is concentrated in the brain, so for specific brain boosting power it is better to choose an oily fish for lunch or dinner.

4. Caffeine
For a quick fix in the morning or afternoon, a cup of coffee should wake you up and increase alertness. More than a couple of cups of coffees a day is not recommended, however, as caffeine is addictive and can do more harm than good if drunk excessively. If you are not a coffee drinker, caffeine can also be found in regular tea, green tea, and energy drinks.

Research has found that around 200 milligrams of caffeine in a mug of coffee is enough to boost brain power and mental alertness. This means that only 2 mugs a day, 1 in the morning and 1 mid-afternoon, are all that are required to improve performance and reduce fatigue.

5. Water

Purely and simply the easiest way to boost brain power is by drinking enough water to stay hydrated. Sluggishness, tiredness, a foggy brain and slow reactions are all signs of dehydration, so just go the tap, drink a glass of water and then take another glassful back to sip at your desk.

It has been said that if you feel thirsty you are already dehydrated, so the best way to keep up hydration levels is to drink between 4 and 8 glasses regularly throughout the day.

Also a mood enhancer, water is an easy choice for a quick brain booster if you have been deprived of sleep or just need a quick, healthy pick-me-up.

Some of these ideas not only have brain-boosting effects, they also offer several other health benefits. Try just 1 each week to see which works best for you and your lifestyle, or incorporate them all into your working week to have a quick and efficient brain that will be running on all cylinders.

TIP 38: WHY WE SHOULD EAT EGGS EVERY MORNING

Eggs have had a hard time in the press, but their misrepresentation is being vindicated by new studies. It has now been shown that eggs do not cause heart disease. In fact, eating eggs actually improves your blood cholesterol levels. Read on to find out why you should add eggs to your morning ritual.

• Eggs can help you lose weight. The balance of protein and fat in an egg is enough to keep you full. That mid-morning snack attack can be a phenomenon in your past. In addition, those who eat eggs for breakfast often make better lunch choices than those whose carb-laden breakfasts are long gone by noon.

• Eggs can improve your memory. Eggs are a dietary source of an essential nutrient called choline. Since our bodies cannot produce enough choline, dietary sources of this nutrient are valuable. Choline has many functions, such as protecting the liver from accumulating fatty tissue. In addition choline is extremely important to brain development. The brain development of fetuses requires plenty of choline, making choline extremely important to pregnant women. Some studies suggest that choline is also important to memory function and may help prevent the memory loss associated with Alzheimer's disease.

• Eggs have all of the essential amino acids. Essential amino acids are those that our body does not make – those we must consume. Sometimes it is difficult for vegetarians to consume the essential amino acids, but eggs can provide an easy, vegetarian solution.

• Eggs can save your eyesight. Two antioxidants found in eggs, Zeaxanthine and Lutein, are important to the retina. This means that consuming eggs can protect the eyes from both cataracts and macular degeneration. In fact, one study revealed that participants who consumed between one and three egg yolks per day increased Zeaxanthine by 114 – 142 percent and Lutein by 28 – 50 percent. These are dramatic results.

• Eggs are priced right. Compared to protein supplements and meats, such as beef, poultry and fish, even free-range, grain-fed, organic eggs are reasonably priced.

• Eggs lower the risk of heart disease. Although eggs contain cholesterol, researchers have concluded that dietary cholesterol does not significantly affect blood cholesterol levels. In fact, the opposite is true. Eating eggs raises your HDL (good) cholesterol while improving the quality of your LDL (bad) cholesterol. Studies have shown that dense LDL cholesterol, along with triglycerides, is the real culprit in heart disease. Eating eggs changes small, dense LDL particles into larger, more buoyant particles that do not clog arteries.

Whether you are hoping to lose weight or add a post workout protein boost to your diet, eggs may be the most natural and cost effective way to enhance your health. Now that the worry about raising cholesterol levels is behind us, we need to help eggs shed their bad reputation. These are nutrient powerhouses that are as close as our refrigerator.

TIP #39: EIGHT SIMPLE WAYS TO EAT BETTER

The thought of dieting can seem daunting. We often associate dieting with deprivation of favorite foods, torturous cravings, flavorless health foods and constant hunger pangs. However, dieting doesn't have to be difficult. It's as simple as incorporating a few simple changes to your lifestyle in a thoughtful way. Here are a few ideas to get your started on your journey toward a healthier lifestyle.

1. **Find healthy foods that you actually enjoy eating.** This may take some time and will require patience and a willingness to test new foods. Likely there are fruits, vegetables, healthy grains and other nutritious foods that you actually like. Once you've found healthy foods that you like, swap out some of your junk food for healthy substitutes. For example, almonds may be a satisfying crunchy snack for those who love potato chips. A juicy peach or bowl of raspberries may be the perfect stand-in for sugary deserts.

2. **Try new recipes to find tasty ways to prepare vegetables.** With the enormous number of recipes available for free on the internet, there are plenty of delicious ways to cook vegetables. Look for recipes that offer flavorful ways to cook vegetables without adding a lot of unnecessary fats. Once you find a recipe that you like, try substituting different types of vegetables to get some variety. For example, a recipe for broccoli may work just as well with cauliflower, green beans, Brussels sprouts or zucchini.

3. **Be aware of portion sizes.** While measuring every food item

is tedious, it may be helpful to measure your portions for a short time to gain awareness of how much you are actually eating. You may be surprised to learn the suggested serving size of some of your favorite foods is a lot smaller than you thought. Once you have retrained yourself in proper portion sizes, you can stop measuring or weighing your food.

4. **Use smaller plates to make your meals look larger.** There are two downsides to using large plates. First, you may accidentally let your portion sizes get out of control. Second, if you are able to keep your portions in check, you may feel like you are depriving yourself when you see a small amount of food on your large plate. Piling a small plate full of healthy foods will eliminate that deprivation message and the lack of room on your plate will help maintain portion control.

5. **Challenge yourself to incorporate more fruits and vegetables into your diet.** A great challenge is to eat two different types of fruits or vegetables at each meal. This is harder than it sounds! But if you are able to find ways to cram your plate full of different types of fruits and vegetables, you will have less room for unhealthy foods. This challenge also gives you the opportunity to try lots of different types of produce, giving you the chance to explore new foods and perhaps find a few new favorites.

6. **Find alternatives to eating out of boredom.** Can't resist mindless munching when watching television? Try sipping some herbal tea instead. Constantly reaching for an afternoon snack while at work? Keep your desk drawers stocked with dried fruit, nuts or sliced vegetables.

7. **Substitute exercise for emotional eating.** Cardio, weight lifting or yoga is an instant mood enhancer. Our bodies release endorphins during exercise so the next time you're a feeling down and tempted to eat an entire carton of ice cream, try excising instead.

8. **Remember, your diet is all about moderation!** Sometimes, we all need to indulge. Giving in to your cravings on occasion is not such a bad thing if you remember to exercise moderation. A single scoop of ice cream, a handful of chips, one slice of pizza or a sugary beverage enjoyed on infrequent occasions can help ease those feelings of deprivation. Just remember to be purposeful in your indulgence: eat slowly to savor your food, keep your portions under control and make sure these indulgences occur infrequently.

Reaching your weight loss goals doesn't have to be about only consuming weight loss shakes and boiled chicken. It is much easier to achieve success when you make your diet about healthy lifestyle changes rather than simply counting calories. Embrace your love of food by searching out delicious healthy foods and recipes. Exercise moderation and allow for the occasional treat. Your slimmer, healthier future is easier to achieve than you may think.

TIP #40: PLANT-BASED PROTEIN VS. ANIMAL-BASED PROTEIN: IS ONE BETTER FOR HEART HEALTH?

Everyone should be concerned about heart health. Heart disease is the number one cause of death in the United States. In fact, about 600,000 Americans die annually from heart disease. While there are many things you can do to lower your risk, such as exercising, not smoking, and controlling your blood pressure, diet also plays a key role in heart health.

Protein is an essential component of a diet. It helps us build and repair body tissue, including your muscles, after a workout. Nine of the 20 essential amino acids necessary for the human health that your body can't make are only found in protein sources.

You can get protein from a multitude of sources. Meat and dairy might come to mind when you think of sources of protein but those aren't the only protein sources. There's a common misconception that plants contain little or no protein but that's not the case. Plants are also a source of protein, but most plants are an incomplete protein source, meaning they lack one or more essential amino acids. You can overcome this shortcoming by eating a variety of plant-based protein sources. For example, you can get a full array of essential amino acids by eating a mixed array of beans, legumes, nuts, seeds, and vegetables. Plus, soy is one plant-based food that is a complete protein.

Still, animal-based proteins are the most common sources of protein in the American diet. These include red meat, poultry, eggs, fish, and dairy products. Plant-based proteins include beans, legumes, nuts, and seeds.

Plant-Based vs. Animal-Based Protein and Cardiovascular Risk
One large study looked at the protein eating habits of more than 80,000 middle-aged women as part of a larger study. The women filled out questionnaires every four years about their eating habits. For 26 years, researchers looked at their eating habits and followed them for evidence of cardiovascular disease.

The results? Women who ate more plant-based sources of protein and dairy had a lower risk of cardiovascular disease than those who ate red meat. The study found that simple substitutions, such as replacing a serving of red meat with a handful of nuts each day, led to a significant drop in cardiovascular risk by as much as 30 percent.

Although fish isn't plant-based protein, the study also showed that switching a serving of red meat for fish reduced cardiovascular risk. According to Mayo Clinic, numerous studies show that plant-based protein may lower cardiovascular risk in the following ways:
- Reduction in cholesterol
- Reduction in bodyweight
- Lowering blood pressure

Processed Meat is the Most Harmful
All meat may not carry the same risks. One study of 134,000 people showed that eating only 5 ounces of processed meat weekly was correlated with higher cardiovascular risks. In contrast, chicken and red meat didn't carry the same heart risk. So, processed meat is the first type of meat to eliminate to lower your risk of cardiovascular disease.

Some studies show a link between consuming red meat and a higher risk of heart disease, but chicken and fish appear to not increase the risk. What makes red meat different? Besides being high in saturated fat, red meat contains lots of iron. You need a certain amount of iron in your diet to produce healthy red blood cells. However, iron can be a pro-oxidant, meaning it causes oxidative stress at higher levels. If you eat a diet heavy in red meat, you're consuming more iron and in a form your body easily absorbs. If your iron stores rise too much, it can be harmful to your liver and heart.

Why Not Eat Both Animal and Plant-Based Protein?
You don't have to consume a vegetarian or vegan diet to get benefits from plant-based protein. As studies point out, substituting plant-based protein for some animal-based protein you eat can lower the risk of cardiovascular disease. Plus, you get additional fiber from plant-based foods that you don't get from animal foods. Here are some ways to add more plant-based protein to your diet:
- Add plant-based protein to your favorite meals
- Cook or order vegetarian once or twice a week
- Swap meat for plant-based alternatives like beans and lentils. Rather than beef burgers, try bean or lentil burgers
- Use hummus instead of mayonnaise
- Eat a variety of different plants including beans, lentils, seeds, nuts, and high-protein vegetables
- Add vegan protein powder to smoothies
- Replace chips and other low-protein snacks with nuts
- Try tempeh as a substitute for meat

It's possible to get enough protein even on a vegan diet but you don't have to go full-out vegan or vegetarian to get the heart health benefits plant-based protein offers. Experiment and you may discover you can be happy with less meat, and you'll be doing something good for your heart.

TIP #41: EXACTLY WHY PROCESSED CARBS CAN BE HARMFUL TO YOUR HEALTH

For many decades, junk science has created one of the worst fads in history: the diet devoid of fat. Ironically, this diet has resulted in heart disease and other complications related to obesity. Gary Taubes wrote two articles explaining why this phenomenon occurs. The first was showcased in Science Magazine in the year 1999. The second premiered in the summer of 2002, in another famous publication. In both of these articles, Taubes explained that fat is not the culprit; in fact, the real culprit is excess carbohydrates. To be more specific, processed carbs can be especially harmful to your health.

Processed carbs can be directly linked to increasing glucose levels within the body. This results in a myriad of consequences, ranging from weight gain to cancer. Dietary fat is actually something the body needs (provided that you consume Omega 3s and polyunsaturated fats). Trans fat is the fat that we want to avoid in a healthy diet, but even that does not equate to the harm caused by carbohydrates.

A plethora of books have been written to explain why excessive carb consumption is bad. Chief among supporters of the no-carb diets is the Atkins Diet. While it remains the most well-known of the no-carb legions, there are several others. The common thread that most no-carb diets share, is the belief that low-fat diets are undesirable. Many studies have already shown direct correlations between low-fat diets and hyperinsulinemia - where glucose levels are abnormally high. This throws off your body's natural homeostasis, and can lead to the need for alternate, less efficient means of energy production. Hyperinsulinemia also causes the body to go through glycosylation - a process that puts one at risk for Alzheimers and other degenerative diseases.

Fortunately, hyperinsulinemia can be avoided by limiting your processed carbohydrate consumption and adhering to consumption patterns that resemble a glycemic index diet. With this diet, you eat foods that will keep your blood sugar at normal levels. As such, your energy level will remain constant, which helps balance your insulin regulators.

According to this diet, foods that have a high glycemic index are considered detrimental. By the same token, foods with a low glycemic index are considered beneficial. The Crossfit Journal offers a list of foods that fall under both categories. In addition to these extremes, there are also "hybrid" foods that lie in the middle of the glycemic index scale. Whole grains and brown rice are a few examples of hybrid carbohydrates, that consumed in moderation, can prove to be beneficial.

Keep in mind that getting off of carbs may not be the easiest thing to do. You will not only feel tired, but you may also suffer with nausea. A bran muffin, or a small bowl of whole grain pasta could be enough to curb these cravings until your next meal. Yes, these choices do not beat a piece of fruit, but they are still better than eating something sugary.

Good food usually includes lean meats, veggies and fruits. The bad foods consist of almost anything processed. Sometimes you might find a few exceptions, but that is not the general rule. Foods that have a high glycemic index tend to be sweet and/or starchy. Basically, if it comes in a box, it is a food you should not consume in large quantities.

The same principle also applies to foods that have a long shelf life. Foods with a high glycemic index tend to last several months - sometimes even years. Conversely, foods with a lower glycemic index last less than a week, as they tend to be fresh perishables. True, this might seem like an oversimplification, but these guidelines will help get you started on a healthy glycemic diet void of processed carbs. Combined with your intense fitness regimen, you'll be well on your way to looking and feeling your best.

TIP #42: FIVE SCIENCE-BACKED REASONS BERRIES ARE ONE OF THE HEALTHIEST FOODS ON EARTH

Whether you're an omnivore, vegetarian, or vegan, berries are a healthy addition to your diet. They have little fat and lots of fiber, vitamins, and minerals that support health. These red and blue orbs are also a tasty addition to any diet. Whether you enjoy them fresh or frozen, berries are a top choice for your health and wellness. Here are five reasons why.

Berries for Brain Health

Blueberries contain considerable amounts of anthocyanins, which provide antioxidant support for brain health. Blueberries also contain copious quantities of an antioxidant called pterostilbene. Early research points to the role pterostilbene may play in reducing age-related cognitive decline.

Many neurodegenerative diseases such as Alzheimer's, Parkinson's, and Huntington's are associated with oxidative stress that causes free radicals to attack the neurons of our brain. Berries contain antioxidants including anthocyanins, quercetin, ellagic acid, and resveratrol that fight oxidative stress, preventing these degenerative diseases by removing free radicals from the brain cells.

While there's no evidence that eating berries can reverse these conditions, they could play a role in prevention.

Heart Health and Berries

Understanding how berries affect the heart is simple. Berries are high in anthocyanins, a class of flavonoids that are powerful antioxidants that protect the heart by neutralizing free radicals that can damage blood vessels and oxidize LDL cholesterol.

Studies also show that compounds in berries improve endothelial function, how blood vessels respond to stress. Healthy endothelial function helps with blood pressure control and may lower the risk of clots forming that can lead to a stroke or heart attack.

Plus, berries may enhance heart health in another way, by their effects on blood lipids. One study found that subjects with insulin resistance who consumed a drink made from freeze-dried strawberries experienced an 11 percent drop in LDL cholesterol, the kind linked with a higher risk of cardiovascular disease.

Benefits for Blood Sugar Control

Several studies show red and blue berries lower the blood sugar response to a meal. Studies that show this were conducted in obese adults with insulin resistance. Being a rich source of fiber and inflammation-reducing compounds, it's not surprising that berries offer this benefit.

Another study found that prediabetics who consumed bioactive compounds in blueberries for six weeks experienced improvements in insulin sensitivity. A bowl of berries can be a satisfying substitute for other desserts that aren't as easy on your blood sugar too.

Berries Are Rich in Vitamin C

If you're looking for a vitamin C-rich berry, choose strawberries. A cup of strawberries has more vitamin C than another popular vitamin C source, the orange. Vitamin C is important for maintaining healthy skin and joints, for wound healing, and for immune health. It's also an antioxidant vitamin that helps protect against free radicals that damage cells and tissues. Humans can't make their own vitamin C, and it's a water-soluble vitamin that gets flushed out of your system quickly. Therefore, you need vitamin C in your diet daily. Berries are an effective way to ensure you're getting enough.

Can Berries Lower the Risk of Cancer?

Berries, particularly blueberries, are rich in phenolic compounds that have potential anti-cancer activity. It's too early to say whether berries have the potential for preventing or treating cancer, but scientists have identified ways in which they could be beneficial:

- Anti-inflammatory activity
- Reduction in oxidative stress
- Reduce DNA damage
- Increased cell death of cancer cells

Scientists are busy exploring these possibilities and will know more in the future. Until then, eat a variety of colorful, whole foods that include berries.

Get the Tasty Benefits

Berries are one of the healthiest foods on the planet, and they're also among the most delicious. As a bonus, they're easy to pack and carry with you while traveling or taking a hike in the woods, and they rank high on the nutrient density scale, the percentage of nutrients per calorie. How can you enjoy their benefits?

Toss them into a smoothie: Berries are delicious and a good source of antioxidants. So why not try adding a couple of handfuls into your next smoothie? They blend well and add a touch of natural sweetness to any smoothie.

Add them to salads: Do you like to top your salad with nuts? Why do that when you can use berries instead? Or you could use both. Berries and nuts are some of the more nutrient-dense plant-based foods you can add to a salad.

Use them in desserts: Desserts are the perfect way to finish off any meal. And since berries are sweet and delicious, they're the perfect ingredient for dessert recipes. Try mixing fresh berries into your banana bread or adding berry sauce on top of your favorite cake. If you're going to eat dessert, make sure it's as nutrient-dense as possible.

Add them to hot cereal: Berries can liven up a bowl of oatmeal with flavor and nutrients. Your morning porridge will have an extra touch of natural sweetness when you add berries. Being smaller in size, blueberries are a tasty and healthy option. And why stop with hot cereal; add berries to regular cereal, too.

Now that you know how nutrient-dense berries are and how to eat them, be sure to add them to your shopping list.

TIP #43: WHY YOU SHOULD AVOID TRANS FATS

This is likely not the first time you have been told to avoid trans fats, as it is one of the worst fats you can consume. The higher the trans fat content you eat, the higher your risk for high blood pressure, high cholesterol, and cardiovascular disease. The Mayo Clinic states that trans fat can raise both your LDL (bad) cholesterol and lower your HDL (good) cholesterol. If you raise the LDL (bad) too much, you are at great risk for heart disease. Here are some things to know about trans fats and why you should avoid them.

About Trans Fats

Trans fats are added to a wide range of foods, mostly those that are not healthy or good for you. It is made in a process called hydrogenation by adding hydrogen to vegetable oil. It is done because it helps the oil spoil a lot slower. Therefore, it is most often used in packaged and processed foods, as it helps to increase the shelf life of these foods, yet they don't feel as greasy. Just by adding the hydrogen to oil increases the cholesterol in the body. Foods with the highest amount of trans fats include baked goods like cookies and cakes, and fried foods, such as French fries and donuts. There are also other fats used in cooking or baking that contain trans fats, like margarine and shortening. Luckily, manufacturers have become aware of the health concerns with trans fats and are starting to use less and less of it in their foods.

Read Your Food Labels

In order to determine what foods contain a lot of trans fats, you should learn to read labels. On the front or back of the label, look for "partially hydrogenated oil." This means hydrogen has been added to vegetable oil, which then converts it into trans fats. This may be on the front of the label or in the ingredients list. When a food does not contain trans fats, it is usually made obvious on the label to encourage healthy shoppers to purchase their food item. On the other hand, the label "complete hydrogenated oil" or "fully hydrogenated oil" does not have trans fats. There may be some trans fats in dairy or meat products, but it isn't as dangerous as processed foods or baked goods.

Dangers of Trans Fats

According to the American Heart Association, having a high LDL (bad) cholesterol level is one of the biggest risk factors for heart disease. Consuming a lot of trans fats can then convert to a high amount of the bad type of cholesterol. The high LDL levels lead to the accumulation of fatty deposits in your arteries, which then stop blood from flowing properly to your arteries. Another harmful effect of trans fats is increasing triglycerides, which is a fat in your blood. This can also cause your arteries to harden. Other dangers of trans fats include leading to inflammation of your blood vessels and fatty deposits of these blood vessels.

Food Recommendations

Aside from reading the labels and avoiding trans fats, it's easy to choose proper and healthy food options that don't contain a lot of this dangerous type of fat. Some oils that are healthy and found in foods as an alternative to trans fats include palm kernel and coconut oil. While these are better than trans fats, they still contain saturated fat, so you should eat these foods in small amounts. The healthiest option is monounsaturated fat, such as what you find in canola, peanut and olive oil. This also includes fish, nuts and other foods with omega-3 fatty acids.

TIP #44: BENEFITS OF PROTEIN SHAKES AND SMOOTHIES

Many people are seeking to increase their intake of quality protein while consuming fewer carbohydrates. Keto, paleo, and many other low-carb diets are encouraging everyone to make these changes. Some people are doing this to reach their weight loss goals while others simply want to feel better or improve athletic performance.

Shakes or Smoothies?

There's no precise line separating shakes from smoothies. Traditionally, shakes were milk shakes and tend to be thicker than smoothies, which are usually made with yogurt. However, you can start your shake or smoothie with anything you want, whether water, juice, milk, or yogurt.

The Convenience of Protein Shakes

Protein shakes and smoothies are useful tools to help you reach these goals. It can be challenging to always eat the optimal diet. It's especially hard when you're out and about during the day, whether at work, school, or even the gym. Protein shakes are a convenient and healthy way to consume nutritious, protein-rich meals during the day. The top benefits of protein shakes are:

- Satisfy your appetite. A protein shake can fill you up while consuming fewer calories than you would in a typical meal.
- Convenient. You can drink a shake in seconds wherever you are.
- Versatile. There's really no limit on what you can add to shakes. You can change up nutrients and flavors whenever you want. You never have to get bored with them.

Choose the Type of Protein

You can use many types of protein to make shakes or smoothies, including:
- Whey
- Casein
- Soy
- Rice
- Pea
- Hemp
- Egg --In addition to adding eggs to your shake, you can find supplements made from egg whites.

Both whey and casein are milk products, while soy, rice, pea, and hemp are plant-based and suitable for vegans or people who are sensitive to dairy. Each type of protein has its own qualities. Whey, for example, is more quickly absorbed by the body compared to casein. If you're looking to get all your essential amino acids, you can get them from whey, casein, soy, pea, and hemp. You also have to consider how you react to different foods. Some people are allergic to soy, for example. You may want to change up your protein source for variety.

What to Add to Protein Shakes
Protein shakes provide a simple way to consume nutrient-rich meals and snacks. In addition to your main protein sources such as whey or soy, you can add many other ingredients for added nutrition. These include:
- Flax seeds
- Chia seeds
- Healthy greens such as spirulina, chlorella, or wheatgrass.
- Oats
- Fruit such as apples, bananas, blueberries, or strawberries.
- Natural sweeteners such as honey, maple syrup, or stevia.

The above are just a few suggestions. You can add your own special blend of ingredients. If you take a variety of supplements, a protein shake or smoothie is a simple way to combine them. Rather than taking dozens of pills or capsules, buy your supplements in powder form and mix them all together. That way, you can ingest everything in one or two servings.

Take Your Protein Shakes Anywhere

You can make protein shakes at home using a blender or mixer. If your ingredients are easily absorbed, you can simply place them in a glass and stir. If you regularly consume protein shakes, a portable shaker makes it easy to mix the ingredients without needing an appliance. You can take your portable shaker with you in the car, keep it at your desk at work, or drink from it before or after your workout at the gym.

Protein Shake Tips to Keep in Mind

It's easy to mix a bunch of ingredients in a blender or portable shaker. However, there are certain guidelines that can help you get more out of your protein shakes.

• Measure out ingredients so quantities match your daily goals. You don't want to add too much or too little protein, for example. You can experiment with different dosages and make changes as necessary.

• Be careful about over-sweetening shakes. This adds calories.

• Experiment with different flavorings for variety. For example, you can add chocolate, vanilla, cinnamon, coconut, and many other flavorings.

• Identify the optimal times to take your shakes. This isn't the same for everyone. Experiment and find out what works best for you.

• Don't overdo it. While protein is a vital nutrient, like anything else you can get too much. Excessive protein can cause medical problems such as kidney stones. Current recommendations are 56 grams of protein daily for men and 46 grams for women. However, that's only an approximation. The amount that's right for you depends on your weight, metabolism, and lifestyle as well as how much protein you get in your regular diet.

Make Protein Shakes Part of Your Healthy Lifestyle
Protein shakes and smoothies can help you enjoy a higher level of health and fitness. However, you also have to pay attention to other important factors. As valuable as smoothies and shakes can be, don't expect them to meet all of your nutritional needs. You also need a certain amount of fiber that's found in solid food. Protein shakes are a good supplement but don't expect too much from them. If you eat a balanced diet and get sufficient exercise and rest, protein shakes can be a valuable addition to your healthy lifestyle.

TIP #45: TOP 5 NUTRITION CONCERNS FOR DIABETICS

The number of people being diagnosed with diabetes is growing faster than any other disease. One in ten Americans already has diabetes and one in four is at risk. Fortunately, the vast majority of diabetics are able to control the disease and improve their outlook with modest changes to their eating habits.

Whether you are diagnosed with diabetes or taking steps to reduce your risk, you should plan a diet where the mix of carbohydrates, protein and fats meets your own personal preferences and health goals. It's important to choose meals that you enjoy in order to stay committed to a healthy meal plan.

Carbohydrates
Monitoring carbohydrates and their effect on blood sugar is the most important aspect of planning diabetic meals. This can be done through carbohydrate counting. With experience, you can estimate the effects of different foods and amounts on your blood sugars.

Fiber
Dietary fiber is important to maintaining blood sugar levels. Ideally, a diabetic will consume 14 grams of fiber for every one thousand calories of food that is consumed. Fiber plays a role in minimizing blood sugar spikes from carbohydrates, so at least half of all grain intake should be from whole grains because they are high in fiber.

Beverages

People who regularly consume sweetened beverages are at greater risk of developing Type 2 Diabetes and have a more difficult time managing their diabetes. Sugar sweetened beverages and fruit juices should be avoided. If you really feel the need to indulge in sugary drinks, the amount should be limited to small portions of fewer than eight ounces and other carbohydrates should be reduced to compensate for the sugars in the beverage.

Alcohol must only be consumed in moderation. Drinking to excess, or drinking in the absence of fibre or protein foods, can cause hypoglycemia and ketoacidosis. Women should not have more than one drink per day; two drinks are the limit for a man.

Fats
Because of the strong correlation between heart disease and diabetes, the consumption of saturated fats should be limited to less than seven percent of total calories. If your diet is 2000 calories per day, saturated fats should be limited to just fifteen grams per day. Trans fats should also be limited because of their tendency to increase the bad cholesterol and decrease the good cholesterol in your body.

Monitoring Health
Diabetics should manage their eating by measuring their blood sugar regularly. When blood sugar is low, they should consume no more than 15 grams of carbohydrate and wait 15 minutes before retesting. If the sugar level is still low then repeat with another 15 grams of carbohydrates, wait another 15 minutes and retest again. Once the blood sugar is raised to a healthy level, eat a healthy snack or meal to prevent the hypoglycemia from recurring.

Diabetics need to pay extra attention to their diet when they are sick. Hormones produced during illness tend to elevate the effect of carbohydrates on blood sugar. When suffering an illness, you should be especially vigilant at monitoring your blood sugar, drink plenty of fluids and refrain from vigorous exercise.

Maintaining a healthy weight is an essential part of diabetic meal planning. Even a small weight loss can substantially reduce the effects of diabetes. Keeping a food diary and monitoring your sugar levels can help you to see how your food choices affect your health, and encourage you to limit unhealthy foods and lose weight.

If you have diabetes, it is essential that you work with your doctor and a dietician to make sure that all your nutritional needs are met. By considering diet choices and monitoring your health carefully, you can substantially reduce the health problems associated with diabetes.

TIP #46: FIVE SURPRISING THINGS IN A CUP OF MATCHA TEA

Matcha is a kind of powdered green tea. It's made by grinding green tea leaves into a fine powder, then whisking it with hot water. Unlike the kind of green tea most people are used to, matcha contains the entire leaf and has a richer, stronger taste.

Traditionally, matcha is served in small cups and drunk in traditional style with a small bamboo whisk, which is used to froth the drink and make it light and foamy. Matcha has been used in Japan for many centuries, but the drink has recently grown in popularity across the world. The finest quality matcha tea comes from Japan.

An Amino Acid that Calms You

If coffee makes you anxious, matcha is an alternative that's less likely to give you the jitters. Matcha contains L-theanine, which research shows has a calming effect on people who consume it regularly. It activates alpha waves in the brain that give you a sense of wakeful relaxation. If you're trying to avoid the stimulant effects of caffeine but still want to drink something that helps you wake up before work or school, then consider a green tea beverage made from matcha powder instead.

More Antioxidants Than Brewed Green Tea

Matcha has more polyphenols than brewed green tea. According to research published in the Journal of Chromatography, matcha has 137 times more polyphenols than regular green tea. Antioxidants fight free radical damage that contributes to aging and chronic health problems like cardiovascular disease and cancer. The polyphenols in matcha tea also have an anti-inflammatory effect that's beneficial for health. Tip: You'll absorb more polyphenol antioxidants from matcha or brewed green tea if you add a squirt of lemon.

Less Caffeine Than Coffee

Matcha contains caffeine, but not as much as coffee. One study found that the L-theanine content of matcha offsets the stimulatory effects of caffeine, so you can drink it at any time of day without worrying about a crash. And remember, matcha isn't just for drinking: Add it to smoothies and baked goods for a boost of antioxidants and flavor.

Vitamin C

Surprisingly, matcha contains significant amounts of vitamin C. A study found that infusions of matcha tea include from 32.12 to 44.8 mg/L of vitamin C. The amount varies with the temperature of the water used to make matcha and the type of matcha. In most cases, the amount of vitamin C in matcha is about double the vitamin C in brewed green tea. Vitamin C is an antioxidant vitamin important for protecting tissues, particularly the collagen that makes up connective tissues, from damage and wound healing. Plus, vitamin C supports immune health.

Potassium

Matcha also contains modest quantities of potassium, a mineral, and electrolyte that helps with blood pressure control. Getting enough potassium helps offset the negative effects of sodium on blood vessels and heart health. The best sources of potassium are fruits and vegetables, but matcha also makes a minor contribution.

The Bottom Line

Matcha is the powdered green tea used in the Japanese tea ceremony, but you don't have to be a monk or a geisha to enjoy this tea. Use matcha as an alternative to coffee or soda. If you're used to drinking coffee or soda with caffeine, switching to matcha will reduce your caffeine intake and give you the energy boost you need without the crash that comes from too much coffee.

Some people even add matcha powder to smoothies or baked goods for more antioxidant benefits. You can find many recipes online for creative ways to use matcha. If you are looking for an alternative to coffee drinks, matcha can be a great choice for you. Enjoy!

TIP #47: EIGHT WAYS TO MAKE DIETING MORE ENJOYABLE

Dieting is a great way to lose weight, tone your body, and improve your overall health. With that said, dieting isn't always great for your mental health. Many people use fad diets or crash diets that end up making them feel drained, depressed, and ultimately losing motivation to diet. Fortunately, there are some effective ways to make dieting more enjoyable.

Cutting down on how much you eat and changing what you eat doesn't have to be unpleasant. In many cases, you can still eat plenty of delicious food each day while still losing weight. Some approaches even allow you to eat your favorite junk foods in moderation. Here are eight of the best ways to make dieting more enjoyable.

1. Learn Some Healthy Recipes
If you're trying to lose weight but you're not a fan of eating plain meals such as tuna and veggies or chicken and rice, find some healthy meals that you love. Dieting becomes a lot easier if you can cut down your calories while still eating delicious meals that you genuinely enjoy.

Healthy food doesn't have to be off-putting. Meals such as grilled chicken stir-fries, chili and lime prawn salads, and pad thai are all easy to make and healthy while still being delicious. You can also make smoothies, yogurt bowls, and all kinds of other tasty treats for breakfast and dessert. There are tons of healthy recipes online, so find some you like and stick to them.

2. Give Yourself A Cheat Day

One of the biggest challenges of dieting is fighting cravings for your favorite foods. Although healthy meals can be tasty and refreshing, sometimes you might miss binging on pizza and cookies. Fortunately, you don't always have to eliminate your favorite junk foods.

Although it's important to cut down on unhealthy, high-calorie meals, you can tackle your cravings by giving yourself a cheat day once a week. A cheat day is a day where you can eat whatever you want. As long as you go back to eating clean and cutting your calories for the rest of the week, you can still stay on track while indulging in some delicious non-dieting foods.

3. Add Some Exercise To Your Daily Routine

Dieting by itself can help you lose weight, but you'll see results much faster if you incorporate some physical activity. You don't have to spend hours in the gym, either. Running, cycling, or even doing some circuits in your home for 20 minutes each day can go a long way. If you want to make exercising even more enjoyable, you might want to find a physical activity that's fun for you. This could be yoga, dancing, martial arts, or even team sports. The great thing about exercising is that it gives you more leeway with your diet. You'll be burning more calories via physical activity, meaning that you can enjoy bigger meals or simply enjoy faster weight loss.

4. Try Intermittent Fasting

Intermittent fasting is an excellent strategy for those who don't enjoy traditional dieting but still want to lose weight. Intermittent fasting usually involves fitting all of your meals into an 8-hour eating window before fasting for the remaining 16 hours of the day. Some people take other approaches, such as fasting for 24 hours after an indulgent cheat day.

As well as helping you avoid cravings, intermittent fasting has many surprising benefits. Fasting helps boost human growth hormone (HGH), increase your metabolism, and even fight off various health problems. It can take some getting used to, but as long as you don't overindulge during your eating windows, using this method can help you lose weight much faster.

5. Drink Flavored Water

Drinking water regularly is one of the best things you can do to lose weight faster. A 2003 study in the Journal of Clinical Endocrinology & Metabolism even found that drinking 500ml of water increases your metabolic rate by 30% in both men and women. That means that simply drinking more water can help speed up your weight loss.With that said, downing half a liter of water isn't always enjoyable. That's why it helps to use flavored water. Flavored water still has 0 calories yet makes drinking water throughout the day more enjoyable. You can even make flavored water yourself by infusing your water with herbs, mints, and other flavorful ingredients.

6. Make Your Meals In Advance

Meal planning can make dieting much more enjoyable. One of the biggest problems that people have with dieting is that constantly cooking healthy meals can become annoying and time-consuming. However, if you plan and make your meals in advance, eating healthy will become much easier.

You might want to set one day aside to make a range of meals for the rest of the week then simply put them in the fridge or freezer to save them for later. If you always have a healthy meal ready to heat in the microwave, you'll be less tempted to head to the nearest fast food joint when you're feeling stressed and hungry.

7. Use A Calorie Counting App To Track Your Progress

Keeping track of everything you're eating each day can be tough. But if you fail to keep track of what you're eating, you could end up overeating and ruining your progress. Luckily, you can now use free calorie counting apps to help you track your progress and stick with your diet.

Apps like Fitbit and MyFitnessPal make it easy to track everything you're eating within minutes and break down your daily calorie intake. In some cases, you might even find that you've eaten less than you need to, allowing you to give yourself a treat. This will make it much easier to stay on track with your diet and ultimately achieve your fitness goals.

8. Drink More Tea

Just because you're dieting and trying to avoid overeating, doesn't mean you have to avoid consuming anything. One of the best things you can do to avoid snacking is to drink more tea. Tea can be incredibly tasty and refreshing as well as helping to boost your metabolism.

A 2013 study in the Journal of Research in Medical Sciences found that drinking four cups of green tea per day led to a significant decrease in body weight, body mass index (BMI), waist circumference, and blood pressure. You can also enhance your tea with healthy additives like lemon, honey, and ginger.

Conclusion

Although dieting can sometimes be stressful and unpleasant, these tips will help make it much more enjoyable. By incorporating these strategies, you'll enjoy the process of losing weight more and might even find that you achieve your fitness goals faster. Try them out for yourself and see how they work for you.

TIP #48: EAT YOUR WAY TO HEALTHY EYES THIS SPRING

Everybody has heard the adage 'eating carrots will make you see in the dark'. Many believe it is an old wives' tale that your nan tells you in order to make you eat your vegetables but carrots are genuinely good for your eyes. Whilst they might not give you the supernatural night vision you dreamed of as a kid, they are stuffed full of beta-carotene (the thing that gives them their orange colour). Beta-carotene is known to slow age-related degeneration and reduce the risks of cataracts. So nan was right – eat your carrots or your eyes may well pay the price.

Carrots aren't the only sumptuous, sight-saving delights out there though. Here are six firm favourites that are good for eye-health and are in season this spring.

1.   Leafy vegetable such as rocket or watercress is the perfect accompaniment to any spring meal. With high levels of vitamin C, these leaves will help to maintain tissue strength and healthy cells. Pair with an oily fish such as salmon or lean meat like chicken for a delicious, healthy meal.

2.   Speaking of oily fish, wild salmon and sardines are just coming into season and are stuffed to the brim with those famous omega-3 fats. Omega-3 helps to protect the tiny blood vessels inside the eye and will keep you seeing your tasty fish for years to come! For best results, steam your fish and serve with fresh salad or vegetables.

3.   Although broccoli is coming to the end of its peak season, it

is still available and can protect the eyes with its high levels of vitamin C. Steam it until tender and it can accompany almost any meal.

4. Kiwi fruit is also packed full of that magic vitamin C and vitamin E – just what you want for eye-health maintenance. It also contains the carotenoid lutein (pronounces 'loo-teen') which will again help protect against that pesky age-related degeneration. It is delicious and easy as a mid-day snack. Just chop the top off and eat the flesh with a spoon!

5. Although eggs don't seem to have a 'season', chickens tend to lay more during the spring because the days start getting lighter and longer but it's still not too hot. Eggs are stuffed full of lutein and another carotenoid zeaxanthin (pronounced 'zee-a-zan-thin'). These carotenoids are primarily found in the retina and lens of the eye, thus offering all-round protection and reducing the risk of cloudy cataracts. Eggs are extremely versatile too – although fried may not be a healthy option, you can poach, bake, boil or scramble them. Just make sure you eat the yolk, because that's where all the goodness is!

6. By far the best spring food for eye-health is spinach. Spinach has no less than four of these fabulous vitamins and minerals that protect your vision: beta-carotene, vitamin C, lutein and zeaxanthin. All these together can help to create a protective lens, shield against light, slow degeneration and protect against age-related illnesses. And it's tasty too! Lay a bed of wilted spinach beneath your sardines or you could even make a refreshing spinach and lettuce soup.

TIP #49: SIX SUPERFOODS THAT HELP BUILD STRONGER MUSCLES

Eating a well-balanced, nutritious diet that is rich in vitamins, minerals, and other key nutrients is essential to increasing your body's muscle mass. For example, protein is composed of amino acids that are a major building block of muscle development, as well as an important source of energy. However, not all sources of protein - like red meat - are healthy when consumed in high amounts. Luckily, protein and other key nutrients are found in a wide variety of common superfoods that are healthy and easy to incorporate into your daily meals.

Here are six superfoods that can help you build stronger muscles - and increase your energy level and endurance when doing physical activities.

1. Chicken
As mentioned, eating high amounts of red meat - like beef - is unhealthy for you. For instance, red meat is high in saturated fat - which can be bad for your heart health. However, chicken is a white meat that is not only healthier than beef, but a rich source of animal protein as well. Therefore, eating chicken can help you build stronger muscle mass, as well as provide you with the energy you need when engaging in physical activities.

2. Eggs
Eggs are another superfood and a good source of healthy protein. Although a majority of the protein is concentrated in the egg white. However, the yolks are rich in vitamin D content.

Vitamin D helps promote normal muscle function.

3. Legumes

If you are looking for a vegetable source of protein, legumes contain high levels of amino acids. Furthermore, they contain lots of magnesium, which can help reduce the risk of muscle cramps.

4. Low-fat Milk

You might not think of milk as being a superfood, but its rich calcium content is a key mineral needed in the development of strong muscles. However, when it comes to drinking milk, you should drink healthier low-fat or skimmed milk options.

5. Spinach

If you are familiar with the cartoon character "Popeye," then you know that spinach is often associated with increasing muscle mass. Spinach is a superfood due to its high nutritional content like vitamin C and glutamine. Glutamine is an amino acid that is critical in the production of muscle mass. In addition to increasing your muscle tone, eating spinach can also provide you with greater endurance when engaging in physical activities.

6. Turkey

Lastly, turkey is another healthy white meat option that is a good source of animal protein. You can eat turkey meat on sandwiches instead of pork-based meats like ham and baloney. Speaking of pork alternatives, turkey bacon is healthier than traditional bacon.

In short, chicken, eggs, and turkey are healthier alternatives to red meat that are high in animal protein content. Legumes are a superfood and a great source of plant-based protein. Drinking low-fat milk can provide your body with the calcium needed to promote good muscle development. Eating spinach can also help you increase your muscle tone and endurance.

TIP #50: COW'S MILK VERSUS SOY MILK: HOW DO THEY DIFFER NUTRITIONALLY?

If you're avoiding dairy due to a milk allergy or lactose intolerance, soy milk is one alternative you might consider. Unlike cow's milk that comes from the mammary gland of a cow, soy milk is plant-based, derived from soy beans. To make soy milk, you first soak soybeans to soften them up and then grind and strain them. You can even make it at home using one of the many soy milk makers available online. The beverage that you get has a texture that's somewhat similar to dairy milk although thinner. Also, the taste is a bit "beanier" than dairy milk, although it's hard to tell the difference when you pour it on cereal in the morning.

Nutritional Differences

Both cow's milk and soy milk are good sources of protein with cow's milk having around 8 grams of protein per serving and soy milk about 7 grams. Cow's milk is higher in carbohydrates, about 12 grams in a serving, while a serving of soy milk only has around 5 grams. Depending upon the brand and whether it contains added sugar, it may be slightly higher than this. If you're trying to watch your carbs, choose a brand without added sugar. Soy milk has around half the fat of cow's milk, 8 grams versus 4 grams.

Chalk one up for soy milk. It has much protein as cow's milk, but fewer carbs and half the fat. Where soy milk falls short is in terms of the micronutrients it contains. We all know cow's milk is a good source of calcium, one cup supplies almost a third of a day's requirements. Unless soy milk is fortified, it's a poor source of calcium and contains no natural vitamin B12, a vitamin found almost exclusively in meat and dairy foods.

Fortunately, you can buy fortified soy milk with calcium, vitamin B12, vitamin D, and other vitamins added back in. In reality, cow's milk is NOT a good source of vitamin D and has to be fortified with this important vitamin most people don't get enough of. If you're using soy milk as a source of calcium and vitamin B12, read the label carefully to make sure the brand you're using is fortified.

The Lactose Issue

One reason people choose to drink soy milk is because they don't consume animal products, but that's not the only one. A significant portion of the population doesn't have enough of the enzyme that breaks down lactose, a sugar found in cow's milk. People suffering from lactose intolerance, as this condition is called, develop cramping, bloating and diarrhea when they consume dairy products in significant quantities. If you fall into this category, you can still drink soy milk since it's free of lactose.

Soy Milk: A Good Source of Isoflavones

Unlike cow's milk, soy milk contains compounds called isoflavones that have weak estrogen-like properties. Some research suggests that the isoflavones in soy may protect against breast cancer, although this is somewhat controversial and still unproven. Some experts have raised concerns that consuming soy products might actually increase your breast cancer risk. The verdict is still out. Drinking soy milk may help lower LDL-cholesterol, the type most strongly linked with heart disease. If soymilk does lower the risk of heart disease, data suggests that you need around 25 grams of soy protein daily to get the benefits, the equivalent of 2-3 cups of soy milk daily.

The Bottom Line

Each type of milk has its advantages and disadvantages. Plus, soy milk is only one of a growing number of non-dairy milk substitutes you can buy at natural food markets. If you've never explored the world of "alternative milks," maybe now's the time to give one a try.

TIP #51: HEALTHY OILS FOR COOKING – KNOW YOUR CHOICES

Consumers have read many reports on the importance of healthy fats in their diet, and the dangers of trans fats. However, many people may find the marketing of these products and range of choices confusing. A closer look at some healthy oils will help you to navigate the complicated range of oils on your supermarket shelves so you can choose those that are highest in monosaturated fats for overall good health.

Olive Oil

Olive oil is probably the best-known healthy fat because of the popularity of the "Mediterranean diet" that is associated with healthier aging and longer lifespan. Olive oil is pressed from the fruit of olive trees and is available in a number of grades. "Extra-virgin" olive oil comes from the first pressing of the olives. "Virgin" olive oil is the second pressing. Third and later pressings may require additional processing to be suitable for use. Olive oil contains both omega-3 and omega-6 fatty acids, phenolic compounds and vitamin E, which are all recommended for good health. However, olive oil is high in calories and should be used sparingly when managing weight.

Canola Oil

Canola oil is pressed from oil rapeseed, a plant that is part of the cruciferous family of vegetables. Canola oil contains omega-3 and omega-6 fatty acids that are necessary for good health, vitamin E and plant sterols. Although high in calories, the calories are from healthy fats that aid in cardiovascular function.

Peanut Oil

Peanut oil imparts a nutty, sweet taste to foods and is low in saturated fat. It contains omega-6 fatty acids, plant sterols, vitamin E and an antioxidant called resveratrol that can help to cut the risk of strokes. Peanut oil is a good choice for deep-frying of foods because it can be heated to a higher temperature before smoking and will absorb less fat into foods.

Flaxseed Oil

Another healthy oil that is often recommended by nutritional experts is flaxseed oil. Though it is a little harder to find, it is worth the effort in terms of nutritional benefit. Flaxseed oil is made from pressing the seeds of the flax plant. The oil is high in omega-3 and omega-6 fatty acids and vitamin E. It may improve cholesterol and cardiovascular health. It may also be helpful in reducing stiffness and inflammation from arthritis. Flaxseed oil can interact a number of medications. You should consult your physician before using it in your daily cooking if you take medication on a regular basis.

Grapeseed Oil

Grapeseed oil, pressed from the seed of ordinary grapes, is high in plant sterols and resveratrol, a health promoting antioxidant, omega-3 fatty acid and omega-6 fatty acid. And vitamin E. It is said to promote healthy cholesterol, good vascular function and can help protect against cancer.

Sunflower Oil

Sunflower oil is made by pressing the seeds of the sunflower. For vitamin E, vitamin B1, magnesium, selenium and manganese, sunflower oil is a good choice. It also contains plant sterols to aid in cardiovascular function and lower cholesterol. It is also high in omega-6 fatty acids.

TIP #52: FIVE SIGNS THAT YOU ARE EATING TOO MUCH SALT

Salt is one of the most common seasonings for dishes around the world. It is found in many foods that people enjoy, mainly crunchy snacks such as chips and popcorn. However, there can be quite a few negative health impacts if you eat too much salt. Here are five symptoms of high salt intake.

Unquenchable Thirst

Feeling constantly thirsty may be a sign that you are consuming too much salt. Water helps to regulate pH levels in the body to prevent dehydration as well as keep organs like the kidneys in good working order. Feeling constantly thirsty may be an indicator that sodium levels in your body are too high.

Edema

Edema refers to the swelling of tissues in the body. The swelling can be caused by several conditions, including liver cirrhosis, kidney disease, nephrotic syndrome, and others. It makes your face and other parts of your body appear swollen and puffy. Also, it may cause pain in your joints. Edema can sometimes occur from consuming too much salt, which causes your body to retain water, appearing swollen and puffy.

Kidney Disease

Kidney disease can result from too much sodium in your body. Excess salt can lead to the formation of protein in your urine. Protein in urine is one of the major causes of kidney disease. High sodium can also lead to the formation of kidney stones, which may cause serious health problems and pain if they are not treated.

High Blood Pressure

High blood pressure is a result of your heart having to pump harder to move blood around your body. If you consistently consume too much salt, more fluid will be retained in your body. As a result, your heart will need to work harder, leading to high blood pressure. Consider reducing your salt intake to avoid this issue.

Headaches

Due to the water retention that results from overconsumption of salt, the volume of blood in your body increases. Your blood vessels are forced to expand to cater for the extra volume of blood. As a result, you can experience frequent and more severe headaches.

In Conclusion

If you notice any of these symptoms, you may need to cut back on consuming salty foods. You may wish to talk to your doctor about your options for reducing your sodium levels. However, you can try introducing other spices into your meals for healthier seasoning options as a starting point.

TIP #53: TOP 5 FOODS FOR
A CLEANSING DETOX DIET

One of the biggest hazards of living in modern Western society is that you are constantly coming in contact with harmful substances through your diet and lifestyle. Although your liver does a great job of keeping your body free of toxins, you can help detoxify your body through eating a diet that is rich in cleansing foods. Here are some of the best detoxing foods that you can eat.

Beets

Beets are one of the healthiest foods that should be a part of your diet regardless of your health goals. They are filling, delicious and packed with vital nutrients such as zinc and magnesium. They may also help decrease your risk of developing cancer. It should be no surprise that this food can also help remove dangerous toxins from your body.

Avocados

Avocados are a fruit that is growing in popularity due to its great taste and ability to complement a wide variety of foods. It is also one of the most nutritious foods that you can eat. Avocados are a good food for detox diets because they contain a very high amount of both soluble and insoluble fiber. Both kinds of fiber are necessary to promote healthy digestion.

Artichokes

Artichokes are another nutrient-rich food that is good for cleansing. It is particularly helpful for people with liver disorders whose bodies have difficulty naturally removing toxins. Artichokes have this effect due to an antioxidant known as silymarin. They also contain a caffeoylquinic acid known as cynarine. This acid allows your body to digest fats more easily.

Dill

Dill is an herb that has been found to promote cleansing. It has a number of vital nutrients and antioxidants. Like artichokes, dill can help your liver work more efficiently. This herb can help your liver by activating an antioxidant known as glutathione. Glutathione helps your liver remove free radicals from your body.

Goji Berries

Goji berries are a superfruit with a number of nutrients and health benefits. They gain their detoxifying properties from their abundance of vitamin C and beta-carotene. Vitamin C is necessary for your body to properly be able to remove waste. Beta-carotene is yet another nutrient that helps your liver perform at optimal capacity.

When it comes to cleansing your body of toxins, the key is to maintain a healthy diet and to take care of your liver. You do not have to stick to a detox diet all year long, but you should aim to fully remove the toxins from your body at least once every few months.

TIP #54: FIVE WAYS THAT RED WINE CAN BENEFIT YOUR HEALTH

Odds are pretty good you've heard that drinking red wine can actually be beneficial to your health - as long as you do it in moderation. But what exactly are those health benefits? The following are 5 of the health benefits that you can be taking advantage of by drinking just one or two glasses of red wine per day:

- **Reduce the risk of heart problems** - There is a strong antioxidant compound in red wine called resveratrol. This antioxidant compound will help to protect your heart against the effects of saturated fat, thereby helping to reduce the risk of heart disease. Red wine also contains saponins and flavonoids, both of which help protect against heart disease. Additionally, alcohol helps to raise your good cholesterol, which is instrumental in helping to prevent blood clots - the leading cause of heart attacks.

- **Reduce the risk of cancer** - Research on the subject has shown that there may be a correlation between drinking red wine in moderation and reducing the risk of cancer. It's believed that one of the antioxidants in red wine, quercetin, might reduce the risk of lung cancer. Researchers also strongly believe that resveratrol can kill cancerous cells. Resveratrol also helps to prevent cancerous cells from removing irradiated particles, which means that resveratrol can make radiation therapy against cancer more effective.

- **Reduce the risk of diabetes** - According to ten years of data collected by researchers at the Wageningen University in the

Netherlands, individuals that consumed red wine had a 40 percent less chance of developing type 2 diabetes than those who did not drink. Researchers believe that this is due to the grapes with which wine is made. Consuming grapes helps to slow down the development of high blood pressure as well as insulin resistance, thereby helping to reduce the risk of type 2 diabetes.

- Prevent cataracts - Several studies have been conducted that have found a link between drinking red wine in moderation and preventing cataracts. When comparing the test subjects, it was found that individuals who either did not drink red wine or were heavy drinkers were 50 percent more likely to develop cataracts than those who drank red wine in moderation.

- Promote healthy teeth - Red wine helps to harden the enamel of your teeth, which in turn helps to prevent tooth decay. You can also help to prevent gum disease by drinking red wine, since it contains polyphenols, which also help to reduce the inflammation in your gums.

These are 5 of the health benefits that drinking a glass or two of wine per day can provide. Just remember that you will only receive these benefits if you drink red wine in moderation. Drinking heavily will eliminate these health benefits as well as cause health problems.

TIP #55: SEVEN PROTEIN-RICH FOODS THAT ARE NOT MEAT

The average American eats about 274 pounds of meat per year. That's more than three times the global average. Plus, people in developing countries are also starting to eat more meat, especially chicken and pork.

Unfortunately, a lot of the meat we eat comes from factory farms, which can raise environmental and public health concerns. Animal waste runs off into rivers and oceans and pollutes them. The sheer number of animals in these places can spread diseases like avian flu or swine flu that then spread to humans. Factory farms also use a lot of energy and water, and produce lots of greenhouse gas emissions. No wonder there's more interest in eating plant-based foods.

If you can reduce your meat intake, you're active in tackling climate change and being an advocate for animal welfare. But what about protein? Plant-based foods also contain protein, and as dietitians point out, you can meet your body's protein requirements without consuming meat. Let's look at some of the best plant-based protein sources that aren't meat.

Tempeh
Although all soy-based foods are high in protein, tempeh is the most protein rich with 15 grams of protein per half-cup. Tempeh is fermented soybeans with a firm texture and nutty taste. With its texture, it's an excellent substitute for meat in dishes like tacos or chili. Soy-based foods are also an excellent source of calcium, magnesium, and some B-vitamins. Plus, because it's

fermented, tempeh may contain probiotics, gut friendly bacteria that support digestive health.

How can you enjoy the benefits of tempeh? To add flavor to this soy-based food, marinate slices overnight in tamari sauce, miso or lemon juice. Use different cooking methods to prepare tempeh. Although you can cook tempeh without any oil by steaming, baking or pan-frying, adding oil will help keep the tempeh from sticking to pans. You can even use oil to fry tempeh if you don't mind the extra calories. Tempeh is delicious when you sear it on a grill too. Enjoy this versatile protein source!

Peanuts

Peanuts aren't a tree nut, but a legume, and they're also packed with plant-based protein. **How much?** A half-cup of these crunchy orbs has 19 grams of muscle-building protein. Plus, studies link a diet containing tree nuts, including peanuts, with a lower risk of cardiovascular disease. Peanuts are also an excellent source of resveratrol, an antioxidant linked with heart health. So, switch those chips for a bag of peanuts. They're a heart-healthy snack.

Lentils

Lentils have almost 9 grams of protein per half-cup serving. They're also surprisingly high in antioxidants. Of all the legumes, lentils rank number two in antioxidant content, just behind black beans, another excellent source of plant-based protein.

How can you enjoy lentils?

•   Serve with quinoa or wild rice with chopped tomatoes and Parmesan cheese.

•   Add lentils to salads for extra texture, fiber, and protein.

•   Substitute lentils for half the ground beef in chili or taco filling. Add to soups or stews for a heartier fare.

•   Make lentil burgers or lentil pancakes.

Quinoa

Although many people think of quinoa as a grain, it's actually a seed and one that's high in protein. A cup of quinoa cooked contains around 8 grams of protein. What distinguishes it from many other plant-based foods, other than soy, is it's a complete source of protein. It supplies all 9 essential amino acids your body needs but can't make.

Quinoa is also rich in fiber, iron, magnesium, and antioxidants. Use it as a substitute for rice, and you'll get more protein and fiber. Raw quinoa is coated with a layer of saponins. Although they aren't harmful, they can make the finished product taste bitter. To remove saponins, rinse quinoa in cold water before cooking.

How can you use quinoa in your own recipes?

- Use quinoa as a substitute for rice.
- Add cooked quinoa to a savory casserole instead of pasta or rice.
- Cook the quinoa and leave it in the fridge overnight to cool down before eating cold in a salad or with vegetables.
- Replace half of the oats in your morning bowl of oatmeal with quinoa. Add nuts and berries.
- Substitute half of the flour in your cookie recipes with quinoa flour for a crunchy texture that tastes delicious.

Seitan

Seitan is wheat gluten with a texture similar to meat. This makes it popular as a meat substitute. It lacks one essential amino acid that needs to be a complete protein, but if you cook seitan in soy sauce, it supplies the missing amino acid, lysine, and makes it a complete protein. A third cup of seitan has a whopping 21 grams of protein, enough to give you a big jump-start on meeting the day's protein needs.

How to enjoy seitan? Add seitan to any meal that requires meat. In a stew or chili, you can crumble in some seitan, add flavor and make part of the dish. But if you want to replicate the feel of meat in your mouth when eating a meal, consider something other than seitan unless you're making an Asian dish.

Hemp Seeds

Although they come from the Cannabis sativa plant, hemp seeds contain only trace amounts of THC, the ingredient in the plant that causes a high. What hemp seeds are better known for is being a good source of plant-based protein. A single ounce has 6.3 grams of protein, along with plant-based omega-3s and fiber.

How can you use hemp seeds? You can eat hemp seeds raw or cooked, and they make a crunchy addition to salad dressings and smoothies. You can also sprinkle them into your morning cup of porridge. The taste is mild and nutty, so it works well with sweet and savory foods. You can even sprinkle them on vegetables for added texture and nutrients.

Black Beans

Popular in Mexican food, black beans are no slouch when it comes to protein. With 15 grams of protein per serving, they'll help you meet your protein needs in a delicious way. Plus, they are the bean highest in antioxidants. Beans are an underappreciated source of nutrients, supplying the body with zinc, magnesium, selenium, and vitamins B1, B6, E, and K. Plus, research links diets high in beans with better blood sugar control and a lower risk of cardiovascular disease.

You probably already know ways to enjoy black beans, but here are some other suggestions:
- Add to soups and stews
- Mix them with garlic, onion powder, or red pepper flakes and

serve as a side dish with rice or corn tortillas
- Make a homemade black bean burger
- Make a spicy bean dip for vegetables.
- Add shredded cheese for a nachos appetizer

The Bottom Line
Hopefully, you have a have a better idea of what you can eat for plant-based protein. It's not so hard to cut back on meat when you have these alternatives. Enjoy!

TIP #56: HEALTHY FOOD ALTERNATIVES FOR MANAGING AND REDUCING STRESS

In the fast-moving and busy world of today, more people are finding stress encroach more into their lives. With these situations and conditions, many people make the choice to ease out their stress by consuming junk food. Since these foods are not ideally suited for high-volume consumption, the amount of calories and sugars contained in them can make people further worse off in terms of their health. However, there are alternative options that can aid in reducing stress while helping you keep a balanced diet. Here are several food options to try if you need a stress-relieving meal.

Foods with Nuts

As stress increases, the amount of B vitamin stores in the body starts to decrease. One of the foods that can help in reversing the decrease in these vitamins is nuts. B vitamins help manage neurotransmitters as well as stress responses such as the fight-or-flight reflex. In addition, nuts contain valuable potassium - this is a nutrient that has shown in research to reduce blood pressure and the effects of stress on the heart.

Red Peppers

Vitamin C is mostly associated with fruits such as oranges, but red peppers carry twice the amount of this nutrient. Studies have also shown that people who consume large amounts of Vitamin C displayed lower blood pressure and recovered faster from physically intensive and stressful activities. In addition, the vitamin C in red peppers can help you lower your cortisol levels - which is a compound associated with the occurrence of stress.

Weekly Salmon Servings

Some of the most important nutrients include Omega-3s. Another study from a mental health magazine indicated that individuals who took daily supplements of Omega-3 had a 20 percent decrease in anxiety. One of the most potent sources of Omega-3 is salmon. By having a weekly serving of salmon, you can maintain more Omega-3s in your body's system. You do not have to search exclusively for salmon for these nutrients, but other types of oily fish as well.

Spinach

Spinach carries a lot of magnesium, which is a valuable ingredient in helping to reduce stress. Low magnesium levels contribute to higher C-reactive protein levels, which can create conditions for higher stress. With added magnesium, you can regulate cortisol and also manage blood pressure. When there is enough magnesium in the body, you can better regulate the elements that are responsible for stress. You can find other primary sources of magnesium in foods such as beans and brown rice.

Oatmeal Plates

Oatmeal is a very comforting breakfast that also helps your brain produce more neurotransmitter serotonin. Additional research from an internal medicine journal indicated that consumers of carbs experience an increased sense of calm. By eating more oatmeal, you can add more complex carbs to your system, which can improve your digestion and also reduce blood sugar. The decrease in blood sugar can correlate with lower levels of stress.

Dark Chocolate

Chocolate cravings can make you reach for a Snickers or Butterfinger bar. However, dark chocolate can help in lowering cortisol levels. Dark chocolate generally contains at least 70 percent of cocoa in their ingredients. The cocoa in dark chocolate can be an important compound in lowering cortisol and stress.

Add Some Tea
Increased tea consumption has been associated with lower cortisol levels. Compared to black tea, the absence of caffeine in decaf and herbal teas helps prevent any elevation in the stress response in consumers. In addition, herbal teas provide relief and a soothing sensation to the digestive tract. Herbal teas help manage stress through the calming of the nervous system within the gut. Chamomile, peppermint, and ginger are helpful tea ingredients that can also help soothe and relax you gut's nervous system.

As more professionals integrate work into their lives, stress becomes more of a common issue. With increased stress, there is a chance you may crave junk food in order to feel better. However, the temporary relief of eating junk food cannot make up for the unhealthy calories and sugars you are adding to your body. By considering and adding alternatives such as tea, oatmeal, dark chocolate, and spinach instead, you can relieve stress-induced food cravings while still maintaining a balanced diet. The next time you experience stress, consider adding these food options to your plans instead of junk food.

TIP #57: SIX REASONS WHY EVERYONE SHOULD BE DRINKING GREEN TEA

Made from the leaves of camellia sinensis, green tea has been used in the east for over 1000 years. Green tea is often praised as the healthiest beverage on the planet. There are dozens of claimed benefits, but how many of them are actually true? Surprisingly, a large amount of them have been backed by scientific research making green tea a very important tool for one's own health.

1) Decreased risk of cancer

Female green tea consumers are 22% less susceptible to develop breast cancer, while men who drink green tea are 48% less likely to develop prostate cancer. For both genders there is a 57% less chance of developing colorectal cancer. One of the main triggers of cancer is oxidative damage to cells. Green tea is full of antioxidant chemicals which can prevent or lessen this damage.

2) Decreased risk of type II diabetes

Increased obesity rates in the first world have led to a much higher prevalence of type II diabetes. Green tea has been shown to reduce blood sugar levels and increase insulin sensitivity, both of which are beneficial for diabetics and those at risk of becoming one. Overall, there is an 18% less chance of developing type II diabetes.

3) Weight Loss

While not directly causing weight loss, green tea contains ingredients that promote weight loss. Polyphenol and caffeine are the main ingredients responsible for this effect. Polyphenol works by increasing the rate of fat oxidation which in turn increases the rate that your body burns calories. Caffeine increases the metabolic rate and increases fatty acid mobilization from the fat cells stored around your body. This increases the amount of energy available and also reduces the size of the fat cells.

4) Improves oral hygiene

Catechins are a type of antioxidant that have been shown to destroy the bacteria and viruses that are commonly found living in the mouth. Green tea can eliminate the bacteria streptococcus mutans, the virus primarily responsible for tooth decay. There is also evidence that catechins can decrease the risk of catching the influenza virus (the common cold).

5) Decreased risk of cardiovascular disease

Green tea reduces the levels of bad (LDL) cholesterol - (low density lipoprotein). High levels of these are the main risk factors for stroke and cardiovascular diseases. Because of the high levels of antioxidants in green tea, the cells in the cardiovascular system are protected from oxidization damage. Green tea has been shown to reduce the chance of developing cardiovascular disease by 31%.

6) Eases Depression

One of the main amino acids present in green tea is theanine. This special amino acid has been proven to provide a soothing and calmative effect on those suffering with depression, increasing the odds of better moods and a heightened sense of well-being.

There are many more benefits of green tea that are yet to be proven by scientific experiments, but until then they remain as theories. Green tea is definitely worth the small price in terms of health benefits. There is no reason that anyone should avoid drinking it.

TIP #58: SEVEN REASONS TO EAT DARK CHOCOLATE EVERY DAY

Chocolate, especially dark chocolate, has been the subject of many scientific studies, and the news for chocolate lovers is simply delicious. To get the most benefit from adding chocolate to your diet, however, make sure to choose chocolate that boasts at least 70 percent cacao. Cacao is more commonly known as cocoa, which is simply cacao that has been roasted and ground.

The goodness of chocolate comes from its cacao concentration. This ingredient contains as many as 300 compounds that provide extreme health benefits, including polyphenols, flavonoids, vitamins, minerals, and healthy fat. Here are just a few benefits you can expect when you regularly consume small amounts of high quality dark chocolate each day.

• **Weight loss.** Yes, you can expect weight loss according to researchers at the University of Copenhagen. These researchers discovered that dark chocolate imparts feelings of fullness. In addition, dark chocolate seems to squash cravings for sweets, fatty foods, and salt.

• **Improved insulin sensitivity.** In addition to being good for your waistline, dark chocolate actually improves insulin sensitivity. Insulin resistance leads to diabetes and metabolic syndrome, but insulin sensitivity leads to a healthy endocrine system and a healthy weight. Some studies even indicate that consuming cacao can prevent diabetes.

- **Happiness**. Similar to exercising, eating dark chocolate raises endorphins, which, in turn, reduce stress. This release of endorphins may be due to dark chocolate's phenylethylamine (PEA) content. PEA is a brain chemical that is associated with the feeling of falling in love. In addition to PEA, cacao also contains tryptophan, an essential amino acid that is used to make serotonin. Serotonin is a neurotransmitter that helps regulate mood. In other words, cacao makes you feel happy. It's an antidepressant.

- **Happy infants.** Pregnant women who ate dark chocolate gave birth to happier babies. This phenomenon is thought to be related to cacao's PEA content. Of course, happier babies lead to happier, less stressed moms, dads, and siblings.

- **Lower blood pressure.** Dark chocolate is loaded with flavonoids, making it a heart healthy food. Those who consume dark chocolate have lower blood pressure as well as improved blood flow. In addition, eating dark chocolate reduces the risk of blood clots.

- **Lower risk of stroke.** Dark chocolate's heart healthy benefits impact more than the circulatory system. Improved blood flow to the brain leads to a decreased risk of stroke.

- **Protection against cancer.** Cacao is full of polyphenol antioxidants. In fact, when tallying polyphenols, cacao trumps the other so-called "super foods," such as blueberries, acai berries, and pomegranates. Polyphenol antioxidants protect the body from free radicals. This protection slows the aging process and even protects the body from cancer and heart disease.

There really is no reason to be afraid of the dark. Dark chocolate can be a healthy addition to almost anyone's diet. Just make sure that you choose chocolate that has plenty of the super-nutrient, cacao. To enjoy the greatest benefits of a little chocolate, choose bars that have at least 70 percent cacao. It has never been easier to eat healthy foods.

TIP #59: FIVE SOURCES OF HEALTHY FAT

Many diets give dietary fat a bad rap. While consuming high amounts of trans fats or saturated fats can certainly lead to health complications and weight gain, moderate amounts of monounsaturated and polyunsaturated fats are essential to a healthy diet, and can even help prevent a host of chronic illnesses such as cardiovascular disease, cancer, and diabetes. Below are some of the best natural sources of these "good" fats:

Nuts

Nuts are a great source of healthy fat, and as an added bonus they contain significant amounts of protein as well. Walnuts, pistachios, and almonds are considered the most nutritionally beneficial nuts, and walnuts have are a great source of omega-3 fatty acids as well. All nuts are rich in vitamins and antioxidants, and increased nut consumption may be linked to lower risks of cardiovascular disease and diabetes. Nut-based butters, such as cashew butter, almond butter, and peanut butter, are another excellent choice.

Vegetable-Derived Oils

While olive oil is rightfully considered the most healthy and beneficial of the cooking oils, other vegetable-derived oils can also be incorporated into a healthy diet. Sunflower oil, peanut oil, canola oil, and coconut oil all have different healthy fat contents, and all can be used with peace of mind. Consumption of these oils has been linked to lower blood pressure and lower risk of cardiovascular disease.

Eggs

Eggs are a great, inexpensive source of both protein and healthy fat. While those with cholesterol issues may need to stick to egg whites, the yolk contains many nutrients, including omega-3 fatty acids and choline, which help keep the brain, heart, and nervous system healthy.

Fatty Fish

Fish such as tuna, salmon, sardines, trout, mackerel and anchovies are an ideal source of protein and dietary fat, and are probably the best way of getting more omega-3 fatty acids in any diet. They also contain plenty of important vitamins and nutrients that help fight off cognitive degeneration, cardiovascular disease, and inflammatory diseases. The American Heart Association recommends at least two servings per week of fatty fish, but eating more than that certainly won't hurt.

Avocado

While avocados are quite high in fat content, weighing in at a hefty 30 grams each, they can also be used as an excellent source of dietary fat in moderation. Avocado consumption has been shown to decrease LDL (bad) cholesterol levels and reduce the risk of cardiovascular disease.

These foods are all ideal sources of heart-healthy polyunsaturated and monounsaturated fats. Diets that incorporate these foods, cut out trans fats, and limit saturated fat intake have been shown to drastically reduce risks of cardiovascular disease, coronary heart disease, stroke, LDL cholesterol, and blood pressure. Switching out less nutritious options for these foods is an excellent first step towards a longer, healthier life.

TIP #60: TEN WAYS TO GAIN HEALTHY WEIGHT

While most Americans are interested in losing weight, many are trying to gain weight. To the surprise of some, gaining weight can actually be a difficult task. Many people try to gain weight by simply eating as much as possible. Unfortunately that can negatively affect your health, so a more refined approach is needed. Here are 10 ways to stay healthy while gaining weight.

Foods High in "Good" Fats

To remain healthy while gaining weight, it is important to look for foods high in healthy fats. Look for foods high in monosaturated fats including avocados, olive oil, sesame oil and canola oil. Avoid saturated fats and trans fats because they can permanently damage the health of your cardiovascular system. Monosaturated fats can lower the risk of heart disease and stroke while helping you gain weight (Heart.org, 2014).

Some nuts also have high levels of monosaturated fat. Macadamias, hazelnuts, pecans and almonds are all extremely nutritious and contain healthy monosaturated fats. Products made from legumes can also be high in healthy fats. Peanut butter is a delicious legume that can help you put on weight. Choose salt-reduced and sugar-reduced peanut butter for a healthier alternative.

Many types of meat are high in monosaturated fats, but they also contain high levels of the less healthy saturated fats. The methods used to cook meat can often introduced additional saturated fats or trans fats, so be careful about how you consume your meat.

Foods High in Protein

Foods that are high in protein can help you develop muscle and put on weight. Some healthier foods that are high in protein include: turkey breast, salt-reduced beef jerky, tuna, salmon, pork loin, pumpkin seeds, lean beef, hard boiled eggs, kidney beans and nuts.

Foods High in Complex Carbohydrates

Complex carbohydrates are very useful for providing the body with energy over longer periods. When combined with protein you have the perfect combination of energy and muscle repair. Complex carbohydrates are often higher in vitamins and minerals than simple carbohydrates such as the ones found in sugar, honey and candy.

Good sources of complex carbohydrates include whole grains, starchy vegetables like potatoes, legumes and green vegetables.

Potatoes are a great addition to a weight-gain diet because they can be easily combined with protein. Add cheese, monosaturated oils, beans, sour cream and meat to your potatoes.

Continue to Exercise

Incorporate a small amount of aerobic activity into your workouts, but focus on building strength. You will notice an increase in your appetite after a good workout, so have a post-workout snack ready. When you add weight in the form of muscle, it persists much longer than adding fat.

Drink Your Nutrients

A great way to increase the amount of calories you are ingesting is by drinking them. Use smoothies that are packed with nutrient-dense ingredients. Some of the best ingredients to use in a weight-gain smoothie include: bananas, flax seed, linseeds, crushed almonds, crushed soya beans, protein powder, milk, mango and avocados. It's important that you don't drink your smoothie before meals, because it can ruin your appetite.

Eat Often

If you are underweight, you will feel full faster simply because your stomach is not big enough to hold large meals. Eat nutritionally dense snacks throughout the day. Buy a small container which you can easily put in your pocket so you can eat while traveling.

Eat Before Bed

The human body's metabolism slows at night, so calories are burnt more slowly. That means more of the calories you consume just before going to bed will add weight. Eat nutritionally dense foods just before going to bed. If you have had a good workout that day, the additional calories will help build muscle while you sleep.

Avoid Packaged Foods

Because you are eating many portions, you should avoid packaged foods with unhealthy ingredients. If you simply gorge yourself on frozen lasagnes you may be eating huge amounts of salt, sugar and trans fats.

Get Scientific!

You can measure the success of your strategy by calculating the total calories you are consuming and your total weight gained. Plan your diet in advance and calculate the total calories for the day, the total vitamins and minerals. Try many different foods to find the most effective for weight gain.

Eat Desert

While the focus is on high-quality protein and complex carbohydrates, there is room for sugar. Eat desert after meals, but try to make it something with at least one positive attribute. For example, a big slice of apple pie covered in fruit and cream will give you extra calories and some nutritional benefit.

By following these simple guidelines, you can put on weight and stay healthy. By concentrating on foods with high levels of nutrients, you will keep your body performing well as you reach your goal weight.

TIP #61: FIVE HEALTH BENEFITS OF CINNAMON

Cinnamon is a spice that is popular for adding flavor to coffee, pastries and other sweet treats. As it turns out, this ingredient also packs quite a few health benefits. Here is a look at some of the healthy effects of consuming cinnamon.

Ulcer Prevention

Contrary to popular belief, ulcers are not caused by stress. The development of an ulcer is related to the presence of a bacteria known as helicobacter pylori. Laboratory research has shown that cinnamon is effective for controlling the population of this bacteria in your stomach.

Cholesterol Regulation

LDL cholesterol is the bad cholesterol in your system. If you have high levels of LDL cholesterol, you are at an increased risk of developing cardiovascular disease and experiencing strokes or heart attacks. Cinnamon has been shown to lower the levels of LDL cholesterol in your body.

Blood Sugar Regulation

Cinnamon has also been shown to regulate your body's levels of blood sugar. Since it helps keep your blood sugar at an optimal level, it is useful for people who suffer from both diabetes and hypoglycemia. It can also help prevent the feeling of crashing after consuming too many simple carbohydrates.

Cancer Prevention

There is some research that indicates that cinnamon might

help reduce your risk of developing cancer. This effect is mostly linked to cinnamon's effect on blood sugar regulation as there is a belief that some types of cancer might be caused by an excess of sugar. There are also specific chemical compounds in cinnamon that can be used to fight colon cancer.

Dental Health

The anti-bacterial properties of cinnamon are linked to improved dental health. Since tooth decay and bad breath are often caused by an excess of bacteria, consuming products that contain cinnamon can reduce your risk of developing these problems. Many brands of chewing gum, toothpaste and breath mints contain cinnamon due to its benefits for dental health.

Cinnamon has a wide variety of benefits for your health and well-being. You should include cinnamon in your diet so that you can experience its rich flavor and enjoy the positive effects that it has on your body.

TIP #62: SEVEN GREAT COMPLEX CARB SOURCES

While many diets try to eliminate or reduce carbohydrate intake, the truth is that not all carbs are created equal. While simple carbs such as processed sugars and syrups can easily be stored as fat, complex carbs are a vital source of energy for the body, especially for those who lead active lives. Incorporating the right carbohydrate choices into a diet is an essential step on the road to better health. Below are some of the most nutritious sources of these complex carbs:

Brown Rice

One of the most common carb sources the world over, brown rice has earned its place as an excellent complex carb. It contains high levels of many nutrients and vitamins, is high in fiber, and can help reduce LDL (bad) cholesterol levels. Brown rice has also been linked to lower risk of many chronic illnesses, including type 2 diabetes and cardiovascular disease.

Beans

Beans come in a dizzying variety of sizes and flavors, but all of them are a great option for adding healthier carbs to any diet. High in fiber and protein, beans are one of the most inexpensive complex carbs, and they can be incorporated into virtually any meal.

Quinoa

A unique, gluten-free grain, quinoa is a complex carb with the added benefit of being a complete protein source, as well. Like brown rice, quinoa contains a variety of useful vitamins and minerals, including essential amino acids. The high protein content in quinoa compared to most other carbohydrate sources makes it an ideal choice for vegetarians or those that lead an active lifestyle.

Fruit

While fruits are technically a simple rather than complex carbohydrate, they earn an exception to the rule due to their many health benefits, as well as the fact that their sugars are naturally-occurring rather than processed. Fruits with lower glycemic content, such as grapefruits, oranges, apples, plums, prunes, apricots, and pears, are generally preferable, but all fruit contains an array of vitamins and nutrients. Berries, in particular, contain relatively high amounts of antioxidants, which help eliminate harmful free radicals.

Sweet Potatoes

Sweet potatoes and yams are both nutritious alternatives to traditional potatoes. They contain high levels of many vitamins, as well as fiber, iron, potassium, and the antioxidant beta-carotene. Regular consumption of sweet potatoes has been associated with decreased risk of diabetes, asthma, and inflammatory diseases.

Oatmeal

Oatmeal makes a wonderful option for breakfast carbohydrate intake. The vitamins and minerals it contains are known to help reduce the risk of stroke, cancer, and cardiovascular disease. Its high fiber content also helps slow digestion and improves nutrient absorption.

Leafy Greens

Leafy green vegetables such as spinach, kale, collard greens, mustard greens, cabbage, and broccoli are some of the healthiest possible carbohydrate options. They contain many vitamins and minerals that are otherwise difficult to obtain, such as calcium, vitamin K, folic acid and beta-carotene. Leafy greens are an inexpensive, low-calorie option that can and should be incorporated into most meals. Consuming high amounts of leafy greens - and vegetables in general - has been shown to reduce the risk of virtually every major chronic illness.

While there are many sources of carbohydrates in the world, it is important to choose the right ones for your health and dietary objectives. These complex carbs can be tailored to fit almost any goal, and incorporating them into any diet is a great way to add variety and ensure that you receive plenty of the nutrients necessary to lead a longer, healthier life.

TIP #63: SEVEN WAYS TO UPGRADE THE HEALTH BENEFITS OF A CUP OF COFFEE

Coffee can be a pick-me-up as well as an excuse to socialize and is a huge part of many people's everyday lives. But have you ever wondered how you can upgrade the health benefits of that steamy cup of hot brew? Studies link coffee drinking itself with possible health benefits. Research shows coffee drinkers may have a lower risk of liver disease, liver cancer, type 2 diabetes, gallstone, depression, and Parkinson's disease. No wonder! Coffee contains over 1,000 compounds including mixtures of proteins, carbohydrates, and lipids, some of which have potential health benefits. So, drinking black coffee is a healthy option to sipping sugar-sweetened beverages. Now, let's discover some ways to make your morning brew even healthier.

Add a Pinch of Cinnamon
Cinnamon has been used in traditional Indian herbal medicine for centuries because of its potent anti-inflammatory properties. Research shows cinnamons lower blood sugar levels while reducing insulin resistance--two factors that directly impact the risk of type 2 diabetes. Plus, a pinch of cinnamon adds delightful flavor and reduces the need for sugar. Get cinnamon from your morning cup of coffee, not a cinnamon bun.

Add a Pinch of Cocoa to Your Coffee Cup
Add a pinch of cocoa to your steaming morning brew. Cocoa contains flavonols, antioxidants that help protect against cardiovascular disease and lower the risk of blood clotting. Plus, flavonols reduce inflammation, another factor that damages blood

vessels and contributes to cardiovascular disease. Cocoa also has modest blood pressure-lowering benefits. And who doesn't enjoy the combination of coffee and chocolate? Choose unsweetened organic cacao powder for the most benefits.

Filter Your Coffee

Filtered coffee is better for your health. You might enjoy a cup of Turkish coffee or French pressed coffee but save it for special occasions. Research shows unfiltered coffee contains compounds that boost blood cholesterol and may increase the risk of cardiovascular disease. When you filter coffee, it removes these compounds and gives you a healthier way to enjoy coffee. In fact, a filtered cup of coffee contains 30-fold fewer of these potentially harmful compounds.

Skip the Sugar

Most people have their morning cup of cofee with cream and sugar, which adds calories and lowers the amount of antioxidant power in each cup. When you add sugar to a cup of coffee, you get a sharp rise in blood glucose. This negates the health benefits of that aromatic cup of coffee that you enjoy during the day. If your coffee needs a hint of sweetness, use Stevia instead. This herbal sweetener has no calories and doesn't trigger a rise in blood glucose like sugar does. It's widely available in many supermarkets.

Avoid Artificial Creamers

If a coffee shop asks if you'd like creamer with your coffee, just say no. The problem with creamers is that many are filled with artificial ingredients that can be harmful. These fake creams are made with ingredients like partially hydrogenated vegetable oils that contain trans fats, and high fructose corn syrup, which ad versely affects your metabolism. A better option is to add a little plant-based milk, like almond or coconut milk, to your morning brew. These days, oat milk is also trendy and they even make barista-style almond milk that froths like dairy milk.

Avoid Artificial Sweeteners Too

Artificial sweeteners might sound like a sweet deal but there's evidence they aren't beneficial for your metabolic health. Studies show that sweeteners in pink, blue, and yellow packs may cause metabolic issues and negatively affect blood sugar control by altering the gut microbiome. Plus, the sweetness of artificial sweeteners does nothing to reduce your desire for sugary foods and beverages. Try slowly decreasing the amount of sweetener you put in your coffee and let your taste buds adapt to less sweet in your life. When you need sweetener, use a natural option that won't affect your blood sugar like Stevia.

Eat Breakfast Before Drinking Your First Cup of Coffee

Studies show the worst time to drink coffee is first thing in the morning. When you first wake up, your cortisol level is at its peak, and coffee can raise it even higher. Cortisol is a stress hormone with negative effects on blood sugar control, body weight, immunity, bone health, and more. After eating breakfast, cortisol starts to come down, so your best bet is to enjoy that coffee after a healthy breakfast that's low in sugar and high in protein.

The Bottom Line

Enjoy your next cup of coffee and make sure you're getting the full health benefits out of each cup you drink.

TIP #64: MANUKA HONEY: WHAT CAN IT DO FOR YOUR HEALTH?

Manuka honey originates from New Zealand and is made from the flowers of the manuka bush. In the last decade has been used as a natural remedy, both internally and externally, due to its antibacterial properties. All honey contains some amount of hydrogen peroxide, an antibacterial chemical, but active manuka honey contains an extra active ingredient that occurs naturally and is known as the 'unique manuka factor' (UMF). A UMF rating is given to the honey and it must be a minimum of 10 as the higher the rating, the more potent and effective it is. You should make sure that you are buying genuine UMF active manuka honey; the Active Manuka Honey Association has issued guidelines that will enable you to check this.

The most common uses of manuka honey are:

Treating wounds
The combination of hydrogen peroxide and the additional properties in UMF manuka honey allow it to not only tackle the infection in the wound, but also to stop any additional bacteria from entering it and to protect from further infection by creating a barrier over the wound. Antibacterial and antifungal properties help to soothe and repair the skin, while the high level of sugar suppresses the growth of micro-organisms.

When manuka honey is used to prevent a barrier between the wound and the dressing, the moist environment speeds up healing, causes less scarring and is less painful. This is because the honey stimulates tissue regeneration and the moist environment means dressing does not stick to the wound, preventing the new skin tissue from being torn away. This application of manuka honey can be used on wounds, leg ulcers and burns and has even been introduced into some hospitals as a method of treatment.

Easing digestive problems

The antibacterial and antibiotic properties can help to fight bacterial infections in the stomach, diarrhoea, indigestion, stomach and peptic ulcers, heartburn and acid reflux. The recommended UMF rating varies depending on what you are using it for, so find out which you need before buying it. For example, UMF 5+ is recommended for maintaining well-being and improving general digestive health and UMF 15+ is for more obvious digestive problems, such as vomiting, ongoing indigestion, diarrhoea or gastric reflux

Sore throats

For centuries, honey has been used as a natural remedy against sore throats and an active manuka honey is even better because of the extra antibacterial properties. Both bacterial and viral infections can cause sore throats, and a streptococcus infection is one of the most common types of bacterial infection. The antibacterial properties in manuka have been found to kill all of the bacteria, including streptococcus.

It is recommended that you take a teaspoon three times a day, holding the honey in your mouth before swallowing it slowly to get the best result. It is a treatment chosen my many because of its pleasant flavour and completely natural origins, with no known side effects (unless you are allergic to honey of course). Other uses for active manuka honey include: fighting gum disease, soothing acne, sunburn and eczema, fighting MRSA (Methicillin-resistant Staphylococcus aureus) infection, providing vocal care and treating cold sores, pressure sores, Athlete's foot, insect bites and arthritis.

The wonderful thing about manuka honey is that it doesn't just have to be used to treat wounds or fight medical conditions; it can be taken daily to promote general health and well-being, and tastes yummy on toast too! If you are feeling creative there are many different recipes you can use it in, so why not give it a try?

TIP #65: HOW TO AVOID MERCURY IN FISH

Nearly every day, there are new headlines proclaiming the health benefits of eating fish. Fish is low in saturated fats and high in protein and heart-healthy omega-3 fatty acids, making it one of the healthiest meats we can consume. Doctors from the American Heart Association recommend eating two servings of fish per week to maintain a healthy diet. But what about mercury poisoning? All fish have trace amounts of mercury in their muscle tissue, so how do we get the benefits of eating fish without the danger of mercury poisoning?

In order to limit mercury consumption it is important to understand how mercury accumulates in the muscle tissue of fish. Mercury is found in the water fish swim in and in the plants and other fish they eat. Fish absorb some mercury from the water, through their gills, however, the majority of the mercury that collects in their muscle tissue comes from the foods they eat. The more mercury-laden food that fish eat and the more they swim in waters contaminated with mercury, the higher their mercury level will be. Mercury never leaves their bodies, so it continues to accumulate throughout their lifetimes.

For this reason, it is wise to avoid older and larger fish. A fish's mercury level increases with every fish it eats. Because older fish have consumed so many other fish throughout their lifetime, their mercury level will be higher than younger fish. For similar reasons, larger fish should be avoided. The larger the fish, the higher up on the food chain it is. A larger fish will have to consume more food, and therefore more mercury, than its counterparts.

There are also certain carnivorous fish that will almost always contain large amounts of mercury. The FDA recommends that shark, swordfish, king mackerel, and tilefish (also known as golden bass or golden snapper) not be consumed by children, pregnant women, nursing women, or those trying to get pregnant. For everyone else, it is safe to consume up to 7 ounces of high-mercury content fish per week. Those concerned about mercury poisoning, however, may wish to avoid them altogether.

So which fish are the safest, in terms of mercury content? According to the American Heart Association the following fish and shellfish have less than 0.1 parts per million of mercury: salmon, catfish, flounder, pollock, shrimp, clams, scallops, crabs, oysters, and herring. Cod, canned tuna, and mahi mahi also contain low levels of mercury.

Eating fish should be a part of your regular heart-healthy diet. Unless you are pregnant, nursing, or a young child, eating up to 14 ounces per week of any kind of fish or shellfish does not put you at risk for mercury poisoning, but if you are particularly concerned about mercury, eat some of the low-mercury fish listed above. The bottom line is: the health benefits of regularly eating fish greatly outweigh the risks of mercury poisoning. So enjoy your tuna sandwich and live a long and healthy life!

BOOKS BY THIS AUTHOR

50 Simple Ways To Eat Better

50 Powerful Exercise Benefits And Tips

130 Reasons Why You Struggle To Lose Weight And How To Fix Them

60 Simple Tips To Stay Healthy And Fit